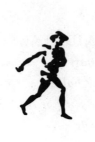

— THE —
PLAGUE
YEARS

A Chronicle of AIDS,
The Epidemic of Our Times

by David Black

SIMON AND SCHUSTER   NEW YORK

Portions of this book have been previously published in
Rolling Stone magazine

Excerpts from *The Normal Heart* © 1985 by Larry Kramer, published by
New American Library, by permission of author.

Library of Congress Cataloging in Publication Data

Black, David, date.
  The plague years.

  1. AIDS (Disease)—Social aspects. 2. AIDS (Disease)—
Popular works. I. Rolling stone. II. Title. [DNLM:
1. Acquired Immunodeficiency Syndrome—history.
2. Acquired Immunodeficiency Syndrome—occurrence.
WD 308 B 627p]
RC607.A26B57   1986   362.1'9697'9200973   86-6481
ISBN: 0-671-61224-7

For Deborah and Susannah

ACKNOWLEDGMENTS

In some cases, I have changed the names of people I spoke with or have left them anonymous. I would like to thank all the scientists, social workers, people with AIDS, and friends who generously gave their time to answer questions and give advice—particularly, Dr. Celso Bianco, Dr. Joel Weisman, Dr. Michael Gottlieb, Dr. Jay Valinsky, Dr. Aaron Kellner, Dr. Steve Witkin, Dr. Joseph Sonnebend, Dr. Max Essex, Dr. Walter Dowdle, Dr. Lawrence Drew, Dr. Mervyn Silverman, Dr. Roger Enlow, the staff of New York City's Gay Men's Health Crisis, Colleen Johnson, Ed Powers, Meg Blackstone and Jeff Moran, Harry Stein and Priscilla Turner.

Larry Kramer, Michael Callen, and Chuck Ortleb gave me an extraordinary amount of time; their help and candor were invaluable.

I would also like to thank Jay Acton once again for all he has done. I must also thank Jann Wenner, David Rosenthal, Bob Wallace, and Cathy Hemming for their support and Susan Murcko and Deborah Bergman for their encouragement and their thoughtful editorial advice.

CONTENTS

He belonged to that race . . . whose ideal is manly precisely because their temperament is feminine, and who in ordinary life resemble other men in appearance only . . . , a race upon which a curse is laid. . . . Their love . . . springs not from an ideal of beauty . . . but from an incurable disease. . . .

—Marcel Proust,
Cities of the Plain

1 / Magna Mortalitas

The period from 1348 to 1352 [the time of the
Black Death in England] is an absolute
blank. . . . Most of the monastic chronicles
are interrupted at the same point; if there is
an entry at all under the year 1349 it is for
the most part merely the words *magna morta-
litas.*

—Charles Creighton,
History of Epidemics in Britain

1.

THE guy by the Baltimore AIDS booth in New York University's Loeb Student Center spread his hand over my note pad.

"You can't do that," he said.

I stepped around him and continued jotting down a description of the exhibit, a cardboard cutout about two and a half feet tall of a condom with a face, chubby little arms and hands, and at the top of his head a nipple, the reservoir tip. In red were the words: *Use me.*

"I said"—the guy put his hands on his hips—"you can't do that."

I looked up from my notes.

"Do what?" I asked.

"Write about me."

"I'm not writing about you," I said. "I'm writing about that."

I gestured at Condom-man.

"I don't believe you," he said.

He craned his neck, trying to read what I'd written. Again I stepped around him.

It was early summer. We were at the Sixth Lesbian/Gay Health Conference, a four-day international convention at-

15

tended by over seven hundred doctors, social workers, sociologists, psychiatrists, psychologists, epidemiologists, sexual ward heelers, acupuncturists, health-food faddists, the sick and the well, the committed and the curious, the angry, the sympathetic, those shocked by the year's events into celibacy and those driven into fatalistic promiscuity.

It felt like a medieval fair. Mingled together among the booths and hawkers were representatives of the different estates. The Lords Spiritual—in the modern world, the keepers of conscience; here, gay and lesbian activists. The Lords Temporal—scientists and politicians. And the Commons— in every era, modern or medieval, the same rank and file. Also present was the class that in a medieval fair would have been represented by the minstrels and fools—the Press—which included me.

And, like a medieval fair, the stink of death was in the air.

Most of what was going on was serious, an attempt to come to grips with gay and lesbian issues, particularly AIDS, the disease that for the few years before the conference had been doubling its victims every six months, mostly in the gay community—an increase that, if it continued at that rate and if it spread into the general population without check, would in a decade kill everyone in the United States and in another decade kill everyone in the world ten times over.

"The good news about that calculation is it makes the threat of nuclear holocaust trivial," said one epidemiologist. "The bad news is that it's only playing with numbers. No disease wipes out everyone."

People were giddy with an anxiety near to joy, the same heightened emotion that comes when you wait for a firecracker to explode or for the midnight countdown to the New Year. I'd seen it when I was a kid during the Cuban missile crisis and when the United States had mined the harbors at Haiphong: the thrill of living on the edge of the apocalypse.

There were workshops on compulsive sexuality, the controversy over bathhouses and bars that offered backrooms for anonymous sexual encounters, organizing AIDS projects in small towns, the communicability of AIDS, safe sex, AIDS and substance abuse, opportunistic infections, and homophobia among doctors and nurses.

There also were pamphlets and newsletters dealing with death, denial, and grief; telling people where to get help, both medical and psychological; and giving descriptions of the early symptoms of AIDS—unexplained fatigue, chills and fevers, night sweats, unexpected weight loss, swollen glands, reddish blue blotches and bumps on the skin, white spots in the mouth, dry cough, diarrhea, and shortness of breath—descriptions that drove people into the bathrooms where in the stalls they nervously checked themselves for telltale signs.

People with unpopular positions, who may have had trouble communicating through official gay organizations, were here able to reach a wider-than-usual audience. Larry Kramer, novelist and playwright and one of the first in the country to organize an AIDS support group, ran a workshop in which he attacked many gay organizations for not demanding enough from the government and distributed an open letter to leaders in the press and gay-rights movement in which he attacked them for failing to adequately inform New Yorkers of the seriousness of the crisis.

The worst epidemic known to modern man is happening right here in this very city [he wrote], and it is one of the best kept secrets around. . . . That all of you . . . continue to refuse to transmit to the public the facts and figures of what is happening *daily* makes you, in my mind, equal to murderers, with blood on your hands just as if you had used knives or bullets or poison. . . . In the name of God, Christ, Moses, whatever impels you to, at last, perform acts of humanity, when will you address this issue with the courage it demands?

One man with AIDS who before he'd gotten sick had spent ten years engaging in backroom sex with, as he described it, hundreds of anonymous partners distributed a position paper, which raised an issue many gays wanted to ignore.

Of those gay "leaders" [it said] who say they are going to bathhouses and backrooms to be an "example" to their brothers that safe sex is possible in such places. I ask you this: How is it possible to have an erotic response when all around you your brothers are engaging in unsafe acts which it is reasonable to assume will result in their deaths? I am told that some S-M practitioners are eroticizing AIDS; that medical scenes [during sex play] have increased—practice for that "inevitable" moment when you will have to "give over control" to your doctor! I'm told that some view AIDS as the ultimate S-M trip: The thought that one might be pumping one's "lovers" full of death—the killer virus—is considered "hot."

"I came here because I needed to talk to others who were sick," said one man with AIDS, who lived in a small Ohio town. "I felt like such a freak when I was a kid because I was gay. Finally, I learned to accept what I was. Be proud of it. And now I feel like a freak all over again because I have AIDS."

At the cocktail party, held at the Institute for International Education on U.N. Plaza the night before the conference began, much of the behavior was inane. One man showed up dressed as a nun. Another looked like Little Bo Peep. A PWA—*Person With AIDS,* which is the politically correct phrase; not *victim, patient,* or even *sufferer*—said, "I want to die with my boots on and my cock out!"

You could tell the PWAs because they tended to be seated, the focus of a constant stream of men who approached and did homage as though death had conferred upon the PWAs authority. They were giving audiences, had become ambassadors from a kingdom beyond the grave.

"Does this look like a crowd capable of fighting for their political or medical rights?" asked one of the founders of New York City Gay Men's Health Crisis.

There were workshops that from their titles sounded ridiculous: *Fat Liberation: A Lesbian Perspective; The Role of [the] Mystical and Magical in AIDS;* and *Feminists Redefine the Clitoris.*

There were conference tote bags and T-shirts with five different designs, gay pride jigsaw puzzles, vibrators, pornographic postcards, specialized books from specialized publishers—like *Anal Pleasure and Health* from the Down There Press—slave bracelets, lots of sickle moons (which suggested some hidden, perhaps unconscious connection between an acceptance of homosexuality and pre-Christian fertility religions) and unicorns (which suggested nothing more than whimsy), a booth promoting spirulina, a blue-green algae touted as "the food of the future," handouts hinting that a macrobiotic diet could cure AIDS, and free copies of *Workers World,* a newspaper that offered a socialist perspective on AIDS. Hybrid organizations, like Gay and Gray and the National Association of Gay Alcoholism Professionals, linked AIDS in a daisy chain of self-help programs.

On every side were examples of the kind of desperate

vanity often found among the old and infirm, an attempt to con Time—and Death.

"We're in a different world," said one gay man. "My mother would die if she saw this."

"I thought of going to psychodynamic theory," said another, "but I read the abstract, and I'm no longer interested."

"That's why I came to this conference," said a third, who was making a circuit of the room, embracing everyone he knew, "to get all these hugs."

There was the usual display of items in questionable taste. A travel brochure plugging the kind of gay bars catering to anonymous pickups in which people can contract AIDS. A throwaway for a Father's Day event, which had a picture of a nearly naked man reading a muscle magazine, his hand inside his jockey shorts, saying, "Cum on, Daddy!" And an advertisement for a "romantic comedy," called *Night Sweat,* which said, "For the ultimate experience, join New York's kinkiest state-of-the-art disco/baths/suicide club. . . . Lifetime membership only $10,000!"

Disco/baths/suicide club. . . .

Even as a joke, it was uncouth. Which was perhaps the point.

Some of the things that appeared vulgar or inane seemed so because they were public expressions of acts or thoughts that, in the straight world at least, are usually private. The academic solemnity, for example, used to discuss the relative risks of various sexual practices didn't jibe with the spirit of the activities involved and inadvertently created the comic effect always produced by the juxtaposition of the high and the low, the formal and the informal. "Anal intercourse insertive versus anal intercourse receptive." *Insertive! Receptive!* What they meant was fucking or being fucked up the ass. The poker-face advice that "Urine on intact skin probably represents little risk" meant: "Don't piss in anybody's wound." And one man in the audience, after a heated panel discussion, responded to a question about the dangers posed by the poor hygiene in bathhouses and on-premises sex bars by saying, "You can't tell where someone's cock has come from? Well, smell it."

Outside the conference hall, visible through plate-glass windows, New York University students sunned themselves on a terrace, oblivious to the passionate exchange about feces, sex, and death.

Such talk in a room set up with the pomp of a presidential news conference does seem surreal. But foolishness, vanity, fatuousness, bad taste, vulgarity, and inanity are not limited to gays. Most cocktail parties and conferences have their share of silliness. And guys arriving at a serious conclave about a fatal disease dressed like nuns or Little Bo Peep are no more outrageous than someone like Simon Eagle, who during the plague of 1664 strode through the streets of London calling down the wrath of God, naked except for—on his head—a pan of burning charcoal.

Outside the student center a hot dog vendor, gazing at a passing gay, waggled a phallic wiener and muttered, "And people worry about getting sick from eating these!"

2.

When I was trying to jot down a description of Condomman, I was hot, tired, and frustrated—at the end of seven months of research and gorged with the horror of everything I had seen and learned. I was not in a generous mood. Not for someone who, because he thought I was writing about him, was determined to get into a fight. Whatever else he was—gay or straight, healthy or sick—he was obnoxious.

I have no idea why he didn't simply walk away. Instead he headed straight at me and, passing, shoved me with his shoulder.

I lost my temper and shoved back.

He knocked the pad from my hands.

This was the kind of petty harassment I've encountered on past assignments in small towns among minor bureaucrats—county clerks who don't want to give out public information and junior high school teachers who during the summer are moonlighting as cops.

I stooped to pick up the pad.

He stepped on it.

"Move your foot, asshole," I said.

He did move his foot—and, in doing so, purposely whacked me in the chin with his knee.

Rearing up, I roared, "You fucking faggot!"

Faggot.

The chatter that had filled the room seemed to die away. And the hundred or so gay men and women in the place seemed to turn in a body toward me.

In retrospect, I suspect, my embarrassment magnified the reaction. Probably a dozen, maybe two dozen people stopped what they'd been doing to look at the jerk who had betrayed his homophobia. I was ashamed.

But even more than ashamed. I was surprised at myself.

Like most men of my generation, I grew up—during the 1950s—at a time when the worst thing you could call another boy was *fairy*—or *sissy, betty, mama's boy, pantywaist, cream puff, powder puff, lily, nance, Miss Molly, queen, pansy, queer, swish, homo,* or any of the other synonyms for *homosexual.*

In the shower after gym class, we studiously avoided even

a glance at each other's genitals. We didn't wear red socks—especially on Thursday, which for some reason was pegged *Queersday*. And of course we never touched one another unless it was with a push or a punch. The closest we ever got to an affectionate—not homosexual, just friendly—hug was a headlock, preferably one that forced the other's face to get red and his eyes to bug out.

There were rumors about certain kids. But the stories were usually vague. Most of us weren't even sure what it meant to be queer. Telltale signs were anything from shyness to excessive acne. Walking funny, of course. Fastening the top button of a shirt. Wearing you pants pulled up to your chest.

Queer wasn't so much a sexual as a social term: it meant strange. Out of it. Alien. It was, I think, an atavistic response. We were Neanderthals looking with suspicion at non-Neanderthals. Romans sneering at the barbarians. Or barbarians sneering at the Romans. Members of one tribe leery of the members of another.

And just as members of a tribe or country or team do when faced with *Others,* we tended to knock the queers. Whoever, whatever they were.

One thing for sure: they weren't tough like us.

So I thought.

The first time I knowingly met someone who was gay was the summer between eleventh and twelfth grade, about four in the morning a couple of weeks after the Fourth of July on Cape Cod on the highway between Hyannis and Provincetown—to which I was hitchhiking, because I'd just read Hubert Selby Jr.'s story "Tralala" in *The Provincetown Review* and that was where *The Provincetown Review* was published. It was also (I'd been told) where all the Beatniks vacationed. And I was trying hard to be a high-school Beatnik, bucking the stereotypes—like Maynard G. Krebbs on "The Dobie Gillis Show" and the characters in the Broadway play *The Nervous Set.*

My parents thought my rebellion "cute" and gave me a parody of the records that help you learn a foreign language, something called *How to Speak Hip,* which had an instructor saying things like, "Like, bring the ax to the short, man, and give me a reefer," followed by a bell, after which you, the listener, were supposed to repeat the phrase. It was funnier than I wanted to admit. But I was too solemn about my rebellion to allow myself to appreciate anything but the Beat canon: Ginsberg, Kerouac, Ferlinghetti, John Clellon Holmes, Selby. . . .

From the books, like *On the Road,* I was learning that the definition of masculinity I'd picked up was not the only one. Sal Paradise and Dean Moriarty were more expressive about their friendship than men were supposed to be—at least according to the schoolyard code of the late 1950s and early 1960s. And from "Tralala" I learned that the schoolyard code's position toward women was not that far from the attitudes that led to the story's gang rape.

I'd also just read Norman Mailer's essay "The Homosexual Villain" in *Advertisements for Myself,* which, although Mailer dismissed it as "the worst article I have ever written" because it was composed "in a state of dull anxiety," had a profound impact on me. In it he described his attitude toward homosexuals as being "the equivalent of a 'gentleman's anti-Semitism,' " and told how he broke through his bias by recognizing that "homosexual persecution [was] a political act and a reactionary act." I thought it was a brave piece. Even then I realized that the courage it took to write it was in direct proportion to the intensity of the prejudice the writing of it had to overcome.

Having embraced what then was an unpopular position—partly, I must admit, because it was unpopular—I was ready, I thought, to embrace a laissez-faire attitude toward gender. People could be whatever they wanted to be, I decided with all the righteous magnanimity of a teenager. Even if they wanted to be, well, *sissies*.

A car squealed to a stop about thirty feet down the highway. I ran through the dark, opened the door, slipped in, and came face to face with a man wearing lipstick and rouge and wearing a sequined evening gown and feathered tiara. His feet, in nylon stockings, were bare. His high-heeled shoes were on the car seat between us.

"Oh, Mary!" he said. "Are you gay?"

I'd never heard the term *gay* before, but I guessed what it meant.

I told him no, and for the next hour listened to his story about how he'd just quarreled with his lover and had left a party to go back to his place in Provincetown. His name was Brian, which obtusely I thought appropriate. According to the playground code certain names were suspect. With his extravagance in dress and speech and emotions, Brian was the stereotype of the fairy. And—the clincher—he was crying.

Men—I knew—didn't cry.

The most they might do—when shattered by circumstance—was to turn away their head and stoically close their eyes for a moment.

But with my baby-Beat opinions, I was willing to accept the guy for what he was—with, naturally, a certain amount of condescension on my part.

At dawn we stopped for coffee.

Brian slipped on his high heels and strode into the diner, which was half-full of truck drivers, Portuguese fishermen, laborers. Tough guys. Guys who—I was sure—never cried. Guys who—I was also sure—were ready to beat the bejesus out of any queer who crossed their path.

Remember: This was in the early 1960s.

If I'd been Brian, I would have been scared to go into the place. Hell, I was terrified to go in with him.

We ordered.

The Tough Guys stared.

Brian didn't blink. Sitting in a booth, he hitched up his dress so he could cross his legs. From his purse he took out a cigar, bit off the end, and lit it.

By the time we'd left and Brian had dropped me off in the center of town, I'd learned a lesson about toughness.

When I got out of college in the late 1960s, I thought I'd left behind the schoolyard code. But here I was, almost two decades later, shouting *faggot!*

The roots of prejudice go deep.

Among the Yahoos—fag-baiters and -bashers—bigotry is predictable. But I didn't expect to find it in myself and my friends. We all considered ourselves enlightened—which reveals how blind we can be to our own folly.

People I know who will storm from a room if anyone uses the terms *nigger, kike, wop,* or calls a woman a *cunt,* regularly use *faggot* and *fag,* both of which are put-downs from their very origin: *fag,* meaning a boy in an English public school who is another boy's servant, often his bum boy. Also: a menial worker. A belittling term that has built-in class contempt. To be a fag implied belonging to a lower order, the social equivalent of being at the bottom of the food chain.

Another possible origin for *fag* also betrays class contempt: *faggot,* a bag of sticks, was a pejorative term for an ugly woman, a whore, and by extension a male prostitute. The "bag of sticks" might also have referred to a less than adequate penis. In its obsolete form, *fag* means "to droop"—a definition that has more than a shade of disdain for what is seen as an unmanly phallus. In this sense it probably derives from *fatigue*—which, in the vicious circle life often makes, is one of the most common symptoms of AIDS.

The first time I heard about AIDS was from a committed radical, an uncompromising defender of civil rights. Tuesday, May 11, 1982. *The New York Times* had just published a major article on the "New Homosexual Disorder," which back then was called GRID, Gay-Related Immunodeficiency.

"One thousand one hundred and sixty!" my friend said. "That's the median number of sexual partners the guys getting the disease have had. Can you believe that? One thousand one hundred and sixty!"

We were furiously peddling on stationary bicycles in a health club.

"Do you know how that makes me feel?" he asked. "I've fucked maybe two dozen, three dozen women in my life. One thousand one hundred and sixty different partners! Good God!"

He was more impressed by the sexual statistic than by the new disease or its fatal consequences.

"If they're fucking that much," he wondered, "when do they have time to get sick?"

We spent the next few minutes joking about what, if we'd stopped to think about it, was a very unfunny subject—which was typical of the reaction of the straight males I knew.

As news of the disease spread, so did the jokes. Most of which were not funny, and many of which betrayed not merely insensitivity but gleeful hostility.

What disease do gay crocodiles get? Gator-aids.

What disease do musicians get? Band-aids.

What disease can you get from kids at a roadside stand? Kool-aids.

How does Anita Bryant spell relief? A-I-D-S.

AYDS—referring to the appetite suppressor: With this, the weight *stays* off.

As AIDS began appearing in other groups: What's the hardest thing about getting AIDS? Trying to convince your parents that you're Haitian.

And three particularly vicious jokes.

What's the medical definition of AIDS? A disease that turns fruits into vegetables.

What does *gay* stand for? "Got AIDS yet?"

A new acronym for AIDS: *WOGS*—Wrath of God Syndrome.

In the media AIDS became a popular subject of fun. In the *Atlanta Journal* Dick Williams ran a column that referred to the risk Mondale might run if he let Jimmy Carter campaign for him: " 'Auds,' or Acquired Unpopular Democrat Syndrome." During his morning radio show on WNBC, Don Imus broadcast a sketch that featured a debate between God and an obviously gay deputy mayor of New York City in which God, hesitating to shake hands, asked the deputy mayor, "You got a surgical glove?" During his HBO performance Eddie Murphy did some AIDS jokes that caused a furor.

"His routine . . . is so sick that I wanted to put my foot through the TV," the New York *Daily News* quoted another Eddie Murphy, chairman of the Christopher Street Gay Festival, as saying. "[It's] unacceptable. We hope to start picketing his personal appearances, shows, and boycott his movies. . . . People are really angry with him about this AIDS routine. He's got to be stopped."

Humor is dialectical. The antigay AIDS jokes were joined by jokes that made fun of the straight public's fear of AIDS and gays.

The political cartoonist Toles drew a man-on-the-street

interview on "What do you think about AIDS?" which researchers at the Centers for Disease Control in Atlanta, one
of the main organizations working on the problem, taped to
a corridor wall outside their office.

"I know it can be fatal," says a gentleman in a porkpie
hat. "I just haven't decided if I think it's serious yet."

"It affects homosexual men, drug users, Haitians, and hemophiliacs," says a woman. "Thank goodness it hasn't
spread to human beings yet."

"If it spreads to the general public, it would be a grave
medical crisis, demanding an immediate government response," says another man.

"And if it doesn't?" asks the interviewer.

The man answers, "It's God punishing homos."

"Good Christian people have nothing to fear," says a
woman, "as long as we stay a million miles away from the
slimy creatures who may have it."

An old lady with her hair in a bun says, "I think it's having a good effect on homosexual behavior, causing them to
be . . . um. . . ."

"Less promiscuous?" offers the interviewer.

"No," she said. "Dead."

"I only hope that scientists are able to discover a cure
soon," says a man with a mustache. "But not too soon."

The *New York Native,* a gay weekly, produced *Gaypoon,* a
humor magazine that was filled with AIDS jokes, including
an interview with a director of the AIDS Task Force at the
Centers for Disease Control who "qualified for his position
by his years of experience as the gossip columnist for *Dance-
gay* magazine."

Bill Misenhimer, the acting director of the AIDS
Project/Los Angeles, called AIDS "Toxic Cock Syndrome."

On her stint as guest host of "The Tonight Show," Joan
Rivers made so many fag jokes that she appeared to be
goofing on a homophobic public. She performed in an
AIDS benefit in Los Angeles. And her catch phrase, "Can
we talk . . . ," has become an often-used tag on literature
aimed at informing gays of the dangers of AIDS.

From jokes to joking graffiti to pure venom. . . . The distance is short. In the men's room of a restaurant near
Hampshire College (which has had a course in AIDS),
someone scribbled [*A male name*] *sucks AIDS victims.* And on
a wall near New York University's Loeb Center, which
housed the Gay/Lesbian Health Conference, was the
scrawl *Gay Rights = AIDS.*

What I realized in the moments after I'd shouted *faggot*
was that any account of AIDS was not just a medical story
and not just a story about the gay community, but also a
story about the straight community's reaction to the disease. More than that: it's a story about how the straight
community has used and is using AIDS as a mask for its
feelings about gayness. It is a story about the ramifications
of a metaphor.

The traditional straight fear that gayness is somehow
catching has found its ideal expression in the equation of
homosexuality with disease: *Gay = AIDS.*

Screw, a magazine that in the midst of its pornography
publishes vicious and sometimes tonic satire, ran a full-
page ad for two bogus products, Fabregay and FabreAids,
"available at fine clubs and discos near you."

> "I fucked two friends, and they fucked two friends, and they
> fucked two friends . . . and so on and so on and so on. Now
> everyone I know has bought it!"

> It's not only catching, it's catching on. Don't you be caught
> dead without it. . . .

The epidemic is not just the disease but the virulent reaction the fear of the disease can release in straights toward gays. And in gays toward straights.

3.

The poles of reaction can be described by two encounters I had while researching AIDS, one at the beginning of my work and one at the end.

The first story.

In August, 1983, when I first started looking into the subject, a friend asked what I was working on.

I was drinking a beer and paused to answer.

He reached over, took the bottle from my hand, and had a swig.

"AIDS," I said.

He spit the beer he'd drunk from my bottle onto my kitchen floor.

The second story.

I was interviewing someone who was dying from AIDS when he abruptly lashed out at me.

"You have no right," he screamed. "No right to do this story."

Ever since starting research, I'd been waiting for someone to make that charge.

"Because I'm not gay?" I asked, ready to argue.

But his answer was not what I'd expected.

"No," he said, "because you're not dying."

2 / Stigma and Stigmata

The leper was by turns the object of vilification and of sympathy. A physician could assure the leper himself that his disease was a sign that God had chosen to grant his soul salvation, but he might simultaneously include in his diagnosis that his patient was morally corrupt. The Church might similarly decree that leprosy was a gift of God, but its bishops and priests would nonetheless use the disease as a metaphor for spiritual degeneration. The leper was seen as sinful and meritorious, as punished by God and as given special grace by Him.

—Saul Nathaniel Brody,
The Disease of the Soul

N March of 1980 a young gay man named Nick came down with an odd, tenacious illness, something like mono: fevers, weight loss, fatigue. . . . The doctors in New York, where he lived, couldn't figure out what was wrong, so Nick's lover flew him from city to city across the country, trying to find someone who could help—without success. By summer they were so desperate that wherever they went they stopped people to ask if anyone had ever heard of anything that caused Nick's symptoms.

When Nick finally died and an autopsy was done, he was diagnosed as having had toxoplasmosis, a disease caused by parasites, *Toxoplasma gondii,* that invade cells and multiply, eventually stretching the cell's walls and creating a pseudocyst or causing the cell to burst like a ripe milkweed pod, sending the parasites out into the system to invade new cells.

Toxoplasmosis rarely makes healthy adults sick. At the worst it might cause a fever and swelling of lymph glands, a mild, possibly unnoticed condition. Only when it infects a fetus can it cause serious brain or eye damage or even death. Severe cases of toxoplasmosis occur in an adult if the immune system, the body's defense against illness, is not working properly.

When one of Nick's Fire Island housemates also came down with a mysterious wasting disease, friends of theirs in the gay community suspected a connection. Sexually transmitted diseases were common, especially among those who had many partners: lice, scabies, urethritis, proctitis, prostatitis, herpes, worms, shigella, campylobacter, amebiasis, hepatitis, and those familiar venereal vaudevillians syphilis and gonorrhea. Rare diseases were appearing all the time, even tropical complaints like lymphogranuloma venereum. Nick and his housemate apparently had gotten one of these new—and serious—bugs. But disease was the sexual tax paid by men who frequented baths and bars with backrooms, where pickups were easy and hygiene was poor.

Like any tax, people didn't relish paying it, would avoid it if they could, but if caught recognized it was something they were foolish to think they could escape. Anyway, science was making progress against many of the sexually transmitted diseases. In fact, there would soon be drugs for hepatitis and herpes. Whatever had hit Nick and his housemate—if it turned out to be anything more than a coincidence—would soon be identified and brought under control.

For those doing a sexual high-wire act, medicine was a safety net.

2.

About the same time—late 1979 and early 1980—Dr. Joel Weisman, a former New Yorker with a private practice in the Los Angeles area, began noticing an increase in the number of patients with a mono-type disease. Weisman had a reputation for being sympathetic to the problems, emotional as well as physical, of gay men, and so lots of gays came to him. He is quiet, methodical, not an alarmist. But this syndrome struck him as odd and potentially dangerous: The patients got fevers and swollen glands and took much longer than usual to get better.

Weisman generally diagnosed the illness as cytomegalovirus, a herpes virus that is common in the United States among slum kids, especially preschoolers, and gay men. The virus, CMV—its initials make it sound like a German luxury car—is excreted in saliva, urine, semen, feces, and possibly breast milk. It is transmitted through what one text calls "close and prolonged contact" and through transfusion of whole blood.

Like toxoplasmosis—the disease Nick was diagnosed as having—CMV usually is so mild it can go unnoticed; and, like toxoplasmosis, it can be particularly severe, even fatal, in someone whose immune system is not working properly. CMV also tends to suppress the immune system—the sicker you are, the sicker you get—creating a whirlpool that can suck you down the drain.

A lot of the men with the CMV symptoms were gay.

In late 1980 one of Weisman's patients, also a gay man, wasn't responding to treatment. For three months he'd been getting weaker. He lost thirty pounds. He ran fevers of around 104 degrees. His lymph glands were swollen. And he developed a yeastlike fungus, called candida or thrush, that caked his mouth, the back of his throat, all the way down his esophagus.

Like toxoplasmosis and CMV, candida usually is not a problem for adults; like toxoplasmosis and CMV, it can be severe in someone whose immune system is not working properly.

"I was stumped," said Weisman. "Before the great advances in medicine in the later part of this century, doctors were essentially documentors of what happened. With this patient, that's essentially all I could do."

3.

In December of that year another physician in the Los Angeles area, Dr. Michael Gottlieb, was studying a patient at UCLA who was suffering from candida. Gottlieb and his colleagues ran some blood tests and found that the man's immune system was in shambles. Eventually the patient was diagnosed as having *pneumocystis carinii* pneumonia.

Like toxoplasmosis, cytomegalovirus, and candida, pneumocystis is often found in infants and people whose immune systems are not functioning properly.

And like Nick, Nick's housemate, and Weisman's patient, Gottlieb's patient was gay.

In March of 1981 Weisman's patient had been admitted to UCLA. Tests showed he had the same immune system abnormalities as Gottlieb's patient. He, too, was diagnosed as having pneumocystis. Within a couple of weeks another of Weisman's patients was hospitalized at UCLA. He'd been suffering from mysterious fatigue and fevers, had been exposed to cytomegalovirus, and had pneumocystis. His immune system was abnormally depressed. And he was gay.

Gottlieb ran across a fourth case of a gay man who'd been exposed to cytomegalovirus and had just died of pneumocystis.

Then, a fifth case: same pattern. Fatigue, fever, cytomegalovirus, pneumocystis, gay.

"I'd like to think we were great scientists," Weisman

said. "We were good observers and had good technical help, and we were at the right place at the right time. Or the wrong place at the right time. New York and San Francisco were seeing cases before us but were not making heads or tails of it."

Weisman and Gottlieb had the advantage because in Los Angeles, Weisman explained, "there are only two major medical schools, compared to seven or eight in New York City." It was easier to see a pattern.

One of the most obvious common denominators was that all five of the patients had used poppers, amyl or butyl nitrite, inhalants that intensify orgasm.

This was Theory One: *whatever the problem was, poppers were the cause.*

The solution: *make poppers illegal.*

"It was at first seen as not a medical but a sociological problem," Weisman said. *"The disco days have gotten some people!"*

There was tremendous resistance, in both the gay and the medical communities, to entertaining the possibility that this might be a new disease.

"We'd wiped out polio and smallpox," Weisman said. Measles, military fever, the "trembles," chlorosis. . . . Wiped out this; wiped out that. He snapped his fingers once, twice, three times. . . .

Medicine seemed to be on the verge of achieving the alchemical dream of a universal nostrum. Even if it came in different forms. Miracle drugs and miraculous technology would save us from—what? Aging? Death? It was one of those things respectable people thought about but didn't discuss. Only visionaries raved about life extension, a geometric increase in medical knowledge that could keep us alive decades beyond the normal life span, so we'd benefit from one breakthrough after another, each discovery giving us the means to extend our lives another few decades so we could be around for the next breakthrough and the next, until nature was forced to betray the very secret of life itself and we had a stranglehold on immortality.

"People had the naive belief that no new killer infectious disease would ever come along," Weisman said. "Then there was Legionnaire's disease, toxic shock, and now this. I've been in practice for fourteen years. My whole generation of physicians up until this time had not had to deal with a disease that could kill the doctor in treatment of the patient. That's why this generation of physicians reacted so terribly."

And why they were so ready to believe in the popper theory. Poppers aren't contagious.

As a theory, Weisman said, "Poppers were an easy out. *This was a disease of the gay community. And you know those gays do all those bad things. They brought it on themselves.*" That sort of reaction. "Even some gay scientists who had very bad self-images looked upon it this way." As for straight scientists, Weisman said, "I remember calling a person [in infectious diseases] to describe what was occurring. He said—and this was a theme very early on—'I don't know what you're making such a big deal of it for. If it kills a few of them off, it will make society a better place.' "

The gay community resisted the idea of a new contagious disease as much as the doctors did. They didn't want to be stigmatized. Sexual lepers. Anyway such a notion seemed preposterous. How could a disease pick out just gays? That had to be medical homophobia.

Most of all a killer infectious disease would put a damper on the fun, the arrival of the fatal guest at the end of Poe's tale "The Masque of the Red Death." And people didn't want anything to interfere with The Party.

No, poppers were the best bet. Little jars with names that

promised a sensation (like Rush) or a macho experience (like Locker Room), sold as a room deodorizer or in tubes that look like miniature party favors, the kind with cardboard tongues sticking out at both ends that kids snap. Sniffed, the chemical dilates blood vessels, making it feel as if you've dropped two Alka-Seltzers into your brain. They're readily available at head shops, newsstands, and specialty shops.

The day before I met with Weisman, I'd bought two bottles of butyl nitrite, brought them back to my hotel room, opened one, and, ready to experiment, instead of inhaling, accidentally poured some down a nostril. I dropped the jar, spilling the rest on the rug, and was lurching back and forth from the sink where I was trying to flush out my nose under a running faucet to the window where I gasped for breath, when room service arrived with dinner.

Wrinkling his nose at the reek from the carpet, the waiter carried the tray to the coffee table. Trying to pretend that it was normal for the skin on the top of my skull to be crinkling like heated Saran Wrap, I snapped on the TV.

"The bubonic plague caused the death of a Kern County man last Friday, according to doctors at the Kern Medical Center," a newscaster was saying.

I switched channels.

On "Buck Rogers" the government was trying to keep secret a new disease that was springing up in cities all over the galaxy.

I snapped off the TV.

The waiter left.

I ducked my face under the cold running water.

So much for direct research on poppers.

I'd bought the poppers at The Pleasure Chest, a kind of sexual Sears that sells whips, chains, studded leather costumes, dildos, feathers, masks—all the gear that conjures up images of human sacrifice on the top of pyramid-shaped temples and makes S-M seem like a debased form of some ancient religion.

The Judeo-Christian tradition has an insecure hold on us: Before it was Christmas Day, December 25 was ancient Britain's *modranecht,* mothers' night; Halloween is the last day of the Celtic year; and the Cupid who decorates our Valentine's Day cards is Eros, son of Mercury and Venus, who uses blood, not water, on his whetstone to sharpen his arrows. Centuries after primitive fertility cults had supposedly vanished, their rites continued to be used all across the Western world, including the United States.

In Missouri—according to *Folklore in America,* an anthology of selections from the *Journal of American Folklore*—a farmer might sow flax by striding naked through the plowed fields before dawn, tossing seeds sometimes into the earth and sometimes at the buttocks of his wife, who was also naked, as they both chanted, "Up to my ass, an' higher too!" And in the silo of a farm my wife and I once rented, we found crucified against the inside walls—presumably as a charm to ensure good crops—the mummified remains of dozens of small animals.

Keeping such information in mind tends to put The Pleasure Chest and the stuff it sells in perspective: It is an eruption of the past into the present, capitalism's exploitation of archetypes.

Although the store's primary orientation is gay, it has straight customers. And its stock—artifacts from the storeroom of our most vicious fantasies—can exercise a dark appeal for the rebellious soul in anyone, gay, straight, polymorphous perverse. . . .

A prohibition, the reason for which we don't understand or admit, is almost a command not only for the stubborn but also for those who thirst for knowledge: we risk an experiment to find out *why* the prohibition was pronounced.

That's from Nietzsche's *The Wanderer and His Shadow*. We have inherited the same Faustian urges that Nietzsche was talking about. We would no more abandon our shadow than Peter Pan did at the beginning of Barrie's play—which is not just a child's tale but also an account of the attractions of paganism. Peter is a diminished version of the Great God Pan, who in the Christian era, with his cloven hooves, woolly haunches, and horns, masquerades as Satan.

The pull of the fast-track S-M gay life, which seems to have been the breeding ground—or at least the staging area—for what increasingly appeared as a new and mysterious disease, is not just a pathology the rest of us can dismiss. Its myths may be buried more deeply in our culture than any of us would feel comfortable admitting. Our civilization—both its sexual and nonsexual customs—often can be reduced to the exercise of power. Check this out with any minority: women, blacks, latins, gays. Check this out in most offices. Check this out in the White House, Congress, and the Pentagon. Check this out in most families—and love affairs. Not just homosexual love affairs. Heterosexual ones, too. It's not merely an amusing coincidence that the object of the modern Western world's first love poems, Petrarch's sonnets, models for six hundred years of romance, was Laure de Sade, an ancestor of the infamous marquis.

The culture in which this disease was apparently first incubated is not something apart from mainstream America: It's mainstream America's Nietzschean shadow.

3 / The Plague Goes Public

In *The City of God* St. Augustine complains of this similarity between the action of the plague that kills without destroying the organs and the theater which, without killing, provokes the most mysterious alterations in the mind of not only an individual but an entire populace.

—Antonin Artaud,
The Theater and Its Double

1.

N the spring of 1981, the five Los Angeles cases of pneumocystis were reported to the Centers for Disease Contol in Atlanta, Georgia, a complex of buildings near Emory University that from the outside looks like a middle-size city's department of motor vehicles. Inside it has the bare, somewhat temporary, low-budget look that government laboratories always had on the 1950s television show "Science Fiction Theater." Its function, however, is anything but low budget.

The CDC was organized in the 1940s to deal with outbreaks of malaria among American soldiers. It was so successful—and fear of some future biological warfare was so rampant—that its mandate was broadened in the 1950s. By the 1980s, when it was reorganized, it had become the epidemiologic equivalent of Wall Street, a federally funded research facility that monitors disease patterns, a center where the country's epidemic highs and lows are charted and where scientific plungers invest in illnesses with good prospects.

It makes sure workplaces are safe, studies the effect of civilization on the environment, through research and fieldwork tries to control the spread of diseases, and trains health workers—medical SWAT teams, ready to immunize and quarantine.

The CDC figured out what causes Legionnaire's disease and toxic shock; it also was involved in the disastrous 1976 attempt to produce and distribute a vaccine effective against swine flu, a medical-political farce that was budgeted at $135 million and that was temporarily stopped when several older people died after receiving the shots.

The first time I visited, around Valentine's Day of 1984, the CDC was bullish on civilian gonorrhea: 14,831 cases for the week. Tuberculosis was weakening: only 395 cases, compared to 442 the previous year at the same time. After a slow start in January, encephalitis was picking up. Mumps, meningococcal infections, and malaria were holding steady.

There had been only 1 case of syphilis in Maine, but 419 in Texas. Fifty-three people had died—from various causes—in Bridgeport, Connecticut; 24 in Gary, Indiana; 66 in Wichita, Kansas; 133 in Nashville, Tennessee; 30 in Ogden, Utah; and 36 in Pasadena, California. One person had gotten the bubonic plague, but no one had gotten anthrax, cholera, or diphtheria.

As for AIDS: The week I visited the yearly total was already up to 257 cases: 1 each in Michigan, Iowa, Delaware, and Oklahoma; 2 in Virginia; 4 each in Arizona and Washington, D.C.; 5 each in Massachusetts and Maryland; 7 each in Connecticut, Ohio, and Florida; 13 in New Jersey; 78 in California; and—121 in New York City.

In an elevator one CDC employee said to another, "I've heard of battered children. I've heard of battered wives. I've heard of battered husbands. But I've never heard of a battered cow. I don't know what that means, exactly."

Battered cow?
Coverage at the CDC is thorough.

2.

The Los Angeles pneumocystis cases were investigated
and written up for the June 5, 1981, issue of the *MMWR*,
the *Morbidity and Mortality Weekly Report,* the CDC's bulletin:
approximately eight hundred words dryly describing the
patients' histories, symptoms, treatment, and fate: two had
died. An editorial note explained:

> *Pneumocystis* pneumonia in the United States is almost exclu-
> sively limited to severely immunosuppressed patients. The
> occurrence of pneumocystis in these 5 previously healthy in-
> dividuals without a clinically underlying immunodeficiency
> is unusual. The fact that these patients were all homosexuals
> suggests an association between some aspect of a homosexual
> lifestyle or disease acquired through sexual contact . . . in
> this population.

As usual, the report was circulated through the CDC's
various departments. Dr. James Curran, then chief of the
Venereal Disease Research Department, read it. *Previously
healthy. Homosexual lifestyle. Sexual contact.*

It wasn't even clear that this—whatever it was—was a
sexually transmitted disease. But it was, Curran thought,
"a very strange" and ominous development, a warning of
the panic that would follow. The next week, at a seminar
on sexually transmitted diseases in San Diego, Curran and
another CDC doctor heard about similar cases of pneumocystis in San Francisco.

By the time Curran got back from the conference, the CDC had learned about similar patients in New York City, some of whom were also suffering from a rare cancer called Kaposi's sarcoma.

3.

Kaposi's sarcoma. KS. In the United States it's a disease of the shuffleboard set. Mostly male—a woman's chance of getting it was 1 out of 10—Eastern European Jews or Italians (who seemed to have a genetic predisposition to it). The kind of complaint that old folks, sunning themselves on park benches, might moan about. The purple blotches: one more aggravation along with gas, spindle-shanks, constipation, and arthritis. The disease typically was not severe. It behaved, as one text said, "in an indolent fashion," seemingly as worn out, even bored, as the men who suffered it. For the average case, the treatment of choice was elastic support socks. And maybe some mild X-rays on the skin lesions.

Like toxoplasmosis, cytomegalovirus, candida, and pneumocystis, Kaposi's sarcoma usually is not a problem for young people whose immune systems are functioning properly.

But the Kaposi's cases in New York were young men. Some also had pneumocystis. Some had candida. Many had evidence of cytomegalovirus.

All were gay.

4.

Curran and Dr. Dennis Juranek, then deputy director of the CDC's division of parasitic diseases, went to New York.

"We saw the [Kaposi's] cases there, read a few charts, came back, and started calling around," Curran said.

Were there many other cases of Kaposi's and pneumocystis? Where were the cases occurring? Were the two diseases connected?

"There was some plausible link between the two diseases from the beginning," Curran said.

By midsummer Curran and his colleagues had learned of twenty-six Kaposi's cases, twenty in New York City and six in California. Six also had pneumonia, which in four was confirmed as pneumocystis. Twelve of the Kaposi's patients had been tested for evidence of cytomegalovirus; all twelve had it.

And all twenty-six men were gay.

The report in the July 3, 1981, issue of the *MMWR* admitted that "the occurrence of this number of KS cases during a 30-month period among young, homosexual men is considered highly unusual. No previous association between KS and sexual preference has been reported."

There was also word of ten new cases of pneumocystis in gay men: four in Los Angeles and six in San Francisco.

And four gay men in New York City had developed such bad cases of anal herpes their anuses seemed to be rotting away. Herpes was another disease that, although a nuisance, was usually not serious. One of the four was infected with cytomegalovirus. All had immune systems that were not properly functioning. Three had already died.

The *MMWR* report warned: "Physicians should be alert for Kaposi's sarcoma, PC [*pneumocystis carinii*] pneumonia, and other opportunistic infections associated with immunosuppression in homosexual men."

The big question was: Is this syndrome contagious?

In the July 3 issue of *The New York Times,* which was one of the first newspapers to pick up the story, Curran was quoted as saying, "The best evidence against contagion is that no cases have been reported to date outside the homosexual community."

The hope was that the syndrome was environmental.

"Perhaps certain homosexuals in certain urban centers have been breathing, eating, drinking, or wearing unusual things, behaving in unusual ways, or frequenting unusual locations," said the *New York Native*, a gay newspaper.

"Subsequent enquiries seem to support the view that Kaposi's sarcoma is associated with traumatic sex," Alexander Cockburn wrote in *The Village Voice*, "or in less elevated parlance, such activities as fist-fucking."

This view outraged many gays, who saw it as an attack on gay liberation, as though a fist thrust up a partner's ass was the equivalent of a fist raised in radical salute.

Cockburn's comment was also disliked because of its medical implications. If fist-fucking was associated with this syndrome, it suggested that the syndrome was catching after all; the agent, whatever it was, entered the bloodstream through internal cuts and abrasions. And that brought the argument back to its starting point: If the syndrome was catching, what was it?

In the *New York Native*, Dr. Alvin Friedman-Kien, a professor of dermatology and microbiology at New York University Medical Center, the man who had contacted the CDC about the New York KS cases and who is considered by many to be the forgotten hero of AIDS research, explained that the relatively benign form of KS found in the United States had a malign cousin in Uganda. The gay baths and backrooms, with their poor hygiene, mimicked the unhealthy conditions of equatorial Africa, in which the fatal form of KS flourished. They were, in a way no one had previously suspected, a sexual third world.

By the end of August the CDC knew of seventy more

cases of pneumocystis and Kaposi's, almost all in men from California and New York who were young, white, and gay.

Forty percent of the patients, a startlingly high number, had died.

5.

Apparently toxoplasmosis, cytomegalovirus, candida, pneumocystis, Kaposi's, and severe herpes infections were only manifestations of some greater problem involving a malfunction of the immune system that allowed otherwise relatively mild diseases to kill. Maybe one of the diseases was the agent screwing up the immune system. Maybe not. The only thing clear was that although the specific ailments could be treated, the underlying problem remained and would lead to reinfection.

"It's the worse way I've ever seen anyone go," said a physician at New York Hospital. "I've seen young people die of cancer. But this is total body rot. It's merciless. A young person, a journalist for a magazine in New York, had cerebral toxoplasmosis from a parasite that will affect normal people, but usually benignly. You've probably had it. I've probably had it. Anyone who has been exposed to cats has probably had it. This guy, very bright, realized he was becoming short of memory. His interests were becoming limited. The deterioration progressed relentlessly until he couldn't carry on his job. While he was in the hospital, he suffered a generalized seizure. Then another, so prolonged he needed anesthesia to prevent his limbs from jerking all over. The body was still because of the drugs, but the brain never stopped seizing."

This was not just a new disease. New diseases are not uncommon—like O'nyong-nyong fever, which first appeared

in humans in 1959; Lassa fever, which made its debut in
1969; and Legionnaire's disease. This syndrome was a different kind of disease, an illness that attacked the body's
ability to defend itself.

And it was spreading. Fast.

There were now more than 180 cases. The syndrome had
been detected in at least one woman and among junkies—
politely called drug- or IV-needle abusers by doctors who
wanted to prove their fairness. They saw themselves as ref-
erees outside the struggle in which The Others, the sick,
were engaged.

Still, most of the patients—at that time about 90 percent—were gay men.

Articles began appearing in the popular press.

*Puzzling new syndrome. . . . Mysterious Ailment Plagues Drug
Abusers, Homosexual Males. . . . New Disease . . . Baffles Scientists. . . . A mysterious new syndrome that turns usually harmless
viruses and bacteria into killers has become a public health haz-
ard. . . . Dramatic Spread. . . . Out of Control. . . . Diseases That
Plague Gays. . . .*

About that time the CDC had fallen on hard times. A
few months after the third *MMWR* report on this mysterious gay-related syndrome appeared, Senator Sam Nunn, a
Democrat from Georgia, the state in which the CDC's main
offices are located, announced, through an aide, that he was
"concerned about preserving the integrity of the CDC's
programs"—which would have to be scuttled if proposed
administration budget cuts were carried out.

In December a CDC official warned that the centers
might be forced to lay off as many as 780 employees; the
staff of the Infectious Disease Branch, the division that
fights epidemics, might be cut nearly in half.

Such cuts, Nunn said, "could present a serious threat to
the health of our nation and the world."

Most of the press-release hysteria focused on the danger
to the program that immunized kids against childhood diseases like polio, measles, and rubella. But AIDS got its
share of publicity. The CDC's office of Public Affairs sent
out a newsletter reprinting an article on Kaposi's, pneumocystis, and cytomegalovirus. Articles appeared in *The New
England Journal of Medicine*, *The Wall Street Journal*, *Newsweek*,
and over the wire services.

The CDC budget ended up being cut less than many had
expected. Its allocation for fiscal year 1982 for the mysterious syndrome that was hitting the gay community was $2
million, part of a total federal outlay of a little over $5.5
million. In 1976 the appropriation to fight the swine flu, an
epidemic that turned out to be a will-o'-the-wisp, was $135
million. But swine flu, the government had thought, threatened everyone; and this disease seemingly threatened only
society's misfits: gays and junkies, groups that didn't have
visible voting blocks.

Two million dollars—what a top baseball or basketball
player can make in a year. Or just six times what the president makes in salary plus perks like his travel and party al-
lowance. People have spent more than that on an
apartment in New York City.

Still, even if the AIDS business was not big business, at
least it was in business.

"It became apparent," Curran said, "we needed an organization."

6.

The office of Dr. James Curran, who was made director
of what at first was called the Kaposi's Sarcoma and Op-

portunistic Infections Task Force, had no windows. In fact, when I visited, there appeared to be no windows in any of the task force offices, which were housed in what gave the impression of being a renovated subway station, a wing of the CDC that according to one source once served as the menagerie, where the laboratory test animals were kept.

By 1985, when the AIDS epidemic had begun spreading with epidemic rapidity, thirty-eight people worked directly for the task force. Another seven were stationed out in the field. And sixty were in various CDC laboratories.

On Curran's wall was a large calendar and a map of the United States: time and space—two crucial factors in any epidemic. On his bookshelf: texts on epidemiology, public health, *The Sex Researchers, Law and Forensic Medicine, Human Sexual Response,* volumes on syphilis, birth control, drug addiction, the environment, Paul Brodeur's *The Expendable Americans, The Gonococcus.* On a file cabinet was the obligatory decoration for the office of any academic, psychotherapist, or scientist, for anyone who wants to advertise a global reach of mind and an aesthetic sense sophisticated enough to appreciate the primitive—two African wood sculptures. One was tall and thin, the other was short and fat, the African sculpture version of Abbott and Costello.

"We wanted to interview as many cases as we could, so we could get some clues," Curran said.

Curran came across efficient and slick, a politician's advance man who is too modest to claim to be important himself but who lets you know how important the cause he's working for is. A kind of I-don't-want-to-be-arrogant-and-rude-but-you-know-what-we're-up-against attitude, forgivable in someone who has to repeat the same story over and over. He talked about demographics, psychological profiles; discussed population pools as if they were interest groups.

"First," he said, "were they [the patients] really gay? How do we know they're gay? The thing that struck me was it was so easy to tell. *All of these doctors seeing these strange diseases. And the doctors could tell they [the patients] are all gay.* Was this a bias in reporting? Were only gay men being reported? Why was it occurring in New York, San Francisco, and Los Angeles? Why not Des Moines, Pittsburgh, and Washington?"

Well, for one thing, Curran realized, gay men wouldn't be so easily recognized in cities where being gay was considered a liability. After all, engaging in homosexual acts was still against the law in twenty-three states and the District of Columbia.

But even if gay men might not be identified in Des Moines, pneumocystis and KS would—and those diseases weren't being reported there.

"It struck us as unusual," Curran said, "that it [the mysterious syndrome] was turning up in such segments of society," among gays and junkies. "That should tell us something."

Gay leaders today complain that the CDC's initial sample was not typical, overloaded with what were at first called *promiscuous* and then, euphemistically, *sexually active* men. The perception that this mysterious disease hit only sex-crazed orgiasts contributed to the public's contempt for those affected—as though the syndrome, like those it affected, wasn't to be taken seriously.

In fact, the CDC, like many physicians and scientists, seemed embarrassed by the gayness of the disease.

"This never would have happened to you guys if you got married," one researcher said to a gay activist who visited the CDC.

"To each other?" the gay activist asked, ready to agree. Gay monogamy would certainly have reduced the number of people with the disease.

"To women," the researcher said.

When I asked Curran to explain exactly what he meant by "intimate contact," the phrase researchers kept using to describe the conditions under which the syndrome spread, he seemed uncomfortable, squeamish. He stammered and glanced anxiously around the room. Maybe it was just a bad day. Maybe his reaction had nothing to do with the turn in the conversation to anal sex.

"People are more frequently receptive anal—" he started to say, but interrupted himself to dodge the question by explaining, "There's not a lot of good data. Theoretically, you're more likely to be receptive anally as you get older and to accumulate more partners as you get older. Many people who have larger numbers of partners have large numbers of insertive partners rather than receptive partners."

That makes sense particularly if you're talking about sexual activity in one evening: Most people can get someone else off more often than they can have an orgasm.

"There's a generation difference in people who restrict themselves to oral sex rather than anal sex," Curran continued—a point disputed by gay men.

"He started making up all these 'facts' from the data as he interpreted it," said one gay critic of Curran.

Other gays feel that Curran is right. There is a generational difference for everyone in our society, and gay sex, like straight sex, has in recent years become rougher and more S-M oriented.

"All these things," Curran continued, "are easy to mix up in risk factors."

He did an unintentional Rodney Dangerfield imitation, shooting out his chin and running a finger around his collar.

7.

Throughout 1982 it became increasingly plain that the disease, whatever it was, was not exclusively a gay syndrome. Other groups began getting it: Haitians, prostitutes, and women who had sex with bisexual males.

At a meeting in Washington of scientists and what Curran called "health decision makers," someone raised the awkward issue that the syndrome needed a new name. It was not just a gay plague or gay cancer or—the name that had caught on—gay related immunodeficiency (GRID). Especially not GRID.

Names have power.

That's why the orthodox of most religions don't write or speak the name of God. If you know my name, you have a hold on my soul. Having his name known destroyed Rumplestiltskin. It is a sign of our soulless times that being famous—*having your name known*—is thought to be one of the best things that could happen to you. Businessmen put their name on oil companies, ice cream, chicken. Politicians put their names on buttons and bumper stickers. And if our own names don't carry enough weight, we wear on a T-shirt or cap someone else's name—Otter Tail Power Company, The Grateful Dead, Mozart, Peterbilt—or a logo that by being so famous dispenses with the need for the actual name: a swan, a pony, a dead sheep—as though it were our tribal totem.

Aside from identifying the disease too closely with gays,

which upset the hemophiliacs and transfusion victims, GRID evoked too many memories of powerless power systems ("The blackout was caused by a failure somewhere in the GRID"), of gratings that looked like prison bars, of traffic jams (GRID-lock).

But what could the syndrome be called?

There are the geographical illnesses. French pox. Spanish pox. Texas fever. Hong Kong flu. African sleeping sickness. Asian flu. Singapore ear. German measles.

The animal complaints. Parrot fever. Hog cholera. Chickenpox. Cow pox. Rabbit fever. Swine flu. Sheep rot. And, of course, cat scratch fever.

Designer diseases. Black plague. White plague. Yellow jack. Rocky Mountain spotted fever. Black lung. Blue babies. Pinkeye. Scarlatina. And the red death.

Dandy fever sounds like it makes you want to wear a waistcoat, white gloves, top hat, and carry a cane. Bright's disease. Staggers. Proud flesh. What you call a disorder affects how the trouble is perceived. Scarlet fever is just a kind of strep, but the name makes it sound demonic.

"People suggested things that were [very] specific," Curran said. "Names that sounded like something from outer space."

Curran thinks it was Don Armstrong, chief of infectious diseases at New York's Memorial Sloan-Kettering Cancer Center, who finally said, "Well, just call it AIDS."

Acquired immune-deficiency syndrome.

AIDS.

It has an almost saintly sound. As though it were the Saint Francis of epidemics.

"It was reasonably descriptive," Curran said, "without being pejorative."

By the time the name made its appearance in the *MMWR* in the fall of 1982, about a year after the CDC had first been alerted to the existence of AIDS, other diseases had joined the list of AIDS complaints: lymphadenopathy (swollen lymph nodes), lupus (a disease whose name comes from the Latin for *wolf,* because one of its symptoms is skin that looks gnawed), other cancers including Hodgkin's lymphoma, Burkitt's lymphoma (which may be associated with Epstein-Barr virus, the cause of mono), and anemia.

The disease, like a vampire, could manifest itself in many forms; and, like a vampire, it seemed impossible to track down. It was out at night, stalking the backrooms of bars and lonely docks, its power lying in its attraction, its seductiveness, in the prey's willingness to surrender. Most of its victims were relatively young; it seemed to draw strength from the strong, leaving them drained. The disease had an almost mythic presence. But it was simply following the classic pattern of a disease that has been introduced to a previously unexposed population, like the Spanish influenza of 1918, which in one year killed 400,000 Americans with an average age of thirty-three. New diseases tend to hit healthy young adults hardest. But, although AIDS followed a traditional pattern, its effect was radical, unprecedented.

8.

The first hint that the syndrome was appearing among Haitians was a case of toxoplasmosis discovered during an examination of a dead man's brain at Jackson Memorial Hospital in Florida. Instead of a healthy pink, the brain was speckled with blue, colored like a mackerel's belly. It was a clue from the grave, as though a zombie, leaving a trail of unwinding gauze bandages and rotting flesh, had come to the hospital's Grand Rounds to pronounce a curse.

An article in *The New York Times* in July of 1982 reported that thirty-four Haitians, most in Florida and Brooklyn, New York, had various diseases that were rare and were associated with AIDS. Along with the case of toxoplasmosis were cases of Kaposi's, pneumocystis, and cytomegalovirus. Almost all of the patients were men.

Why Haitians? And if Haitians, why not Dominicans, who share the same island. Theories ranged from speculation about voodoo—which can involve ritual scarring of the skin and cutting the flesh (often with dirty knives), injections of various substances that would have a hard time passing FDA standards (like goat's milk), and arcane uses of mixed animal and human blood—to a suspicion that the syndrome was common on the whole island but that the Dominican Republic had a better tourist bureau.

The disease scared off tourists to Haiti, two-thirds of which were Americans. In the winter of 1981 to 1982, seventy thousand Americans visited Haiti; the following winter, the season after the CDC's *MMWR* report on Haitians and AIDS, only ten thousand Americans went. Cruise ships stopped going to Port-au-Prince. According to a *New York Times* report, when one American returned from Haiti, the customs officer was so freaked about the possibility of catching AIDS, she said, "Open your passport. I'm not touching it."

Since tourism was the second largest source of income in Haiti, AIDS—or at least fear of AIDS—caused a disaster. The drop in tourism led to food riots—around the same time the government banned all opposition political activity, a repressive measure typical of the regime of President-for-Life Jean-Claude Duvalier, who was rumored to be gay and suffering from AIDS. Haiti may be the place where the first revolution due to AIDS occurs.

In the Carrefour section of Port-au-Prince, which may be

the most densely populated area in the Western hemisphere, the poverty is so abject, people sell bits of charcoal a few inches long, which they've combed from fires. Displayed on a piece of cloth, the charcoal sticks look like severed fingers. The food in the Carrefour tends to be badly prepared and poorly cooked: *griot,* fatty burned pork, and *cabrit,* underdone goat that tastes like fetid washcloths.

The houses—huts, really—all jumbled together, look like a cubist painting of a slum. Kids, dressed in rags, play in the dust. Adults shuffle along the alleys, dead-faced and stoic. Down the center of the slum runs a stream that is used as a toilet, for bathing, and for cooking water.

In 1975 I went to the Carrefour to research an article. I stayed with a *houn'gan,* a voodoo priest, whose powers had been studied at a parapsychology laboratory in the United States. By Carrefour standards this voodoo priest was a Rockefeller. He even had a gasoline-powered electric generator, which ran a tiny refrigerator in which he made ice—using water from the stream.

My first night there, he wanted to honor me, his American guest, so with all the ceremony of a wine connoisseur presenting me with some hundred-year-old Château Lafitte, he took out a bottle of Coca-Cola, opened it, and poured an inch or so in our glasses—over ice that contained what looked like fecal matter. To refuse the drink would have been a mortal insult, so I gulped it as quickly as I could, before the ice had a chance to melt very much. Everyone in the family had bowel trouble. Now, so did I. At night, even though I was the third to get to the chamber pot (which was passed from room to room in a hierarchical order; to be third was also an honor, like being seated at a banquet above the salt), it was always full. Given my experience with Haitian hygiene, it didn't surprise me when Haitians were added to the list of AIDS risk groups.

On the main road from the Carrefour to the center of Port-au-Prince are the big whorehouses, like the Club Social Cabaret, which are surrounded by massive walls. Inside are compounds with bars, shady groves, and little hovels that the girls and boys use. In these "social clubs," for the price of a blowjob in Manhattan, $25 to $50, you can do virtually anything with virtually anyone: male and female, children and crones.

Such freedom offers not a test of sexual prowess but of the imagination. What do you want? A thimblejob, an around-the-world, the rear-admiral, the python dance, a rum-desire, the Macao sling—which involves two chickens and some piano wire.

Haiti had been a favorite vacation spot for American gays. Maybe the American gays picked up AIDS from male Haitian prostitutes. Or, as the outraged Haitian government suggested, maybe American gays introduced AIDS into Haiti.

But, in *The New York Times* article of July 1982, twenty-three of the thirty-four Haitians with AIDS who were asked denied being homosexual. Only one Haitian admitted using IV drugs. It would also turn out that in Haiti more women had AIDS than in the United States: 20 percent, as compared to 5 percent.

If the Haitians weren't gay and weren't junkies, why were they getting a disease that had seemed to be limited to gays and junkies?

The answer could lie in genetics. It could be coincidence. Maybe, as Antonin Artaud suggests in *The Theater and Its Double,* plagues—AIDS just as surely as the Black Death— are eruptions into civilization of some spiritual force that creatively disrupts society, a disease that "takes images that are dormant . . . and suddenly extends them into the most extreme gestures," something that "reforges the chain between what is and what is not. . . ." And Haiti, with its extremes of poverty and magic, feces and voodoo, is a natural gate through which such a force could enter our world. The Carrefour, like the gay baths, are carnivals in the root sense of the word: celebrations of the flesh before flesh is gone; *carne vale,* "farewell, meat"—not just the orgiastic revel before the asceticism of Lent, but life as a saturnalia before the endless abstinence of death.

Artaud calls plague "a summons of the lymph," a kind of biological Pied Piper, using a compelling music to lead a particular population, those who are attuned, out of this world and into another, which promises to be a land of total satisfaction and turns out to be a mean existence of exile, longing, and death.

Civilization began with shelter: the first cave. And civilized men and women sit safe in their homes, ignoring—or at best watching through picture windows—the uncanny storms outside, the conflict of forces civilization can't explain. Sigmund Freud said that of the three great world systems, "the animistic (mythological), the religious, and the scientific, . . . animism . . . is perhaps the most consistent and the most exhaustive, the one which explains the nature of the world in its entirety."

Civilization has traded safety—protection from dread—for understanding. Science can't explain everything, maybe can't explain the connection between Haitians with their animistic mythology, their voodoo, and other people with AIDS: gays, prostitutes, junkies, the sexually promiscuous—all of whom have in one way or another smashed the picture window protecting them from the storm and let the uncanny winds roar into the room.

Maybe to solve the puzzle of why certain people get a

disease and others don't, why, as Artaud said, "the plague strikes the coward who flees it and spares the degenerate who gratifies himself on the corpses," why Haitians get AIDS and Dominicans don't, we need to entertain the mystical and find the link between Haitians and gays with AIDS not in their common tendency to suffer from hepatitis B but in their common tendency to conjure up those dark forces science holds at bay by pretending they don't exist. Certainly being possessed by a *loa,* a voodoo spirit, is not too different from being possessed by the kind of lust that compels someone in a gay bath to have dozens of sexual encounters in a single night. We may need to look beyond science—or at least beyond traditional science—to behavioral medicine, the study of the relation between the mind and the body, between attitude and health.

Tension, anxiety, stress can impair the immune system and make someone vulnerable to disease. Do the gays who get AIDS tend to be more conflicted or feel more guilty about their sexual orientation than gays who don't get the disease? The past, with its judges who condemned behavior we think we have come to accept, is a Fifth Columnist within our minds that affects our attitudes in ways that might appall us. Consciously we may resist the pull of the Puritans that tends to make Americans wary of all eroticism, let alone homoeroticism. The more at odds with the past we become (and in the last quarter of the twentieth century, Americans, gay and straight, are very at odds with their past), the more furious the fight between the Fifth Columnist and our conscious minds. To protect ourselves from such psychic civil war, we might be tempted to annihilate the past—which, of course, cannot be done without annihilating the present and the future as well. AIDS is a pretty good annihilator.

Is a population, such as the one in Haiti, that is suffering under extreme poverty—the worst in the Western hemisphere—and a brutal dictatorship (conditions bound to cause severe stress) more susceptible to AIDS than a population on the same island that lives in somewhat better circumstances? A study done by researchers at UCLA and published in *Science,* the journal of the American Association for the Advancement of Science, suggests that rats who cannot escape from electrical shocks retreat into "learned helplessness," which has been associated with a lowered immune response and, in certain stress-related cancers, increased tumor growth. If hopelessness is immunosuppressive, certainly the victims of a mad-dog dictatorship might tend to have suppressed immune systems—and be vulnerable to the AIDS-type diseases that can take advantage of such a state.

But how do you treat such a disease? Write a prescription for a changed society? Take two Molotov cocktails and call me in the morning?

Better to stay inside the shelter, windows closed and curtains drawn, reading medical textbooks and stropping Ockham's razor.

The simplest explanation for the connection between Haitians and gays may be in human nature.

Among such a desperately poor people as Haitians, a man who prostitutes himself may not consider himself to be homosexual: He is merely doing what he can to provide for his family. Also, in Latin cultures you are not considered gay if you are the active partner in a homosexual encounter, so it is possible that a Haitian may have been having gay sex without considering himself gay. The taboo against homosexuality is so powerful that maybe some of the Haitians, prostitutes or not, simply lied. Asking someone in

Port-au-Prince if he sucks cock is not the same as asking someone on Christopher Street.

It was finally reported in a study published by *The New England Journal of Medicine* that of sixty-one Haitians with AIDS, a "disproportionate" number of them came from the Carrefour, which was "recognized as the principal center of male and female prostitution in Haiti." The study acknowledged the "very strong bias" against homosexuality in Haiti and admitted that many of the Haitians with AIDS may have lied. It recognized that there may be a hidden link between the Haitians who got AIDS and the American gay community. If Haitian men with AIDS were either closet gays who felt a need to keep up a heterosexual front, secret bisexuals, or male prostitutes who sold themselves to gays, they could have given AIDS to their girlfriends and wives, which would explain the larger proportion of women with AIDS in Haiti.

9.

"For every man with a full-blown case of AIDS," said Dr. Joyce Wallace of St. Vincent's Hospital in Greenwich Village, New York, one of the first doctors to treat AIDS, "there are at least ten, probably more, with cases of lymphadenopathy," a persistent swelling of the lymph nodes that may be either a herald of AIDS or a symptom of a mild case.

In the spring of 1982 a prostitute whose boyfriend was a drug addict came to Joyce Wallace. The woman had been hooking for seven years and had had a lifetime total of fifteen thousand sexual partners, both paid and unpaid. She'd had what the report delicately called *oroanal intercourse* with about 20 percent of her clients. That is, every year she licked the assholes of about seventy-two strangers. She hadn't been feeling well lately.

It turned out she had a number of AIDS-associated diseases, including candida, herpes, and pneumocystis. And, like the gays with AIDS, she had an abnormally depressed immune system.

Some of her friends, also hookers, came to Dr. Wallace, who welcomed the chance to examine them to see what could be learned about the relationship between sexual activity and AIDS. Two other hookers also turned up with similar immune system abnormalities.

Wallace wanted to look at a larger sample of hookers. The New York City Department of Health was doing a study of prostitutes to see how many had a new kind of penicillin-resistant gonorrhea. City health workers were going into brothels and asking the hookers for their blood; all Wallace wanted was an extra tube, "just ten cc's," she said, for her research. Hookers get stranger requests.

Twenty-five women agreed to the experiment. All denied using IV drugs. Of course, they were talking to city officials. And even though the program had, as Wallace said, "a hands-off policy with the police," the women may have been unwilling to be candid about use of hard drugs.

Two of the twenty-five had abnormal immune system functions. One woman's system was severely depressed.

"She had a thirty-pound weight loss during the previous year," Wallace said. "She looked ill. She could barely move."

A year later the first hooker returned to Wallace's office for a free checkup. She was much better, had gained some weight.

"The problem with studying women who are prostitutes is you have no control over whether or not they are drug addicts or whether or not their johns are drug addicts,"

Wallace said. "So we have this muddying, contaminating factor, because we know that the sexual partners of drug addicts are at risk of getting this disease."

By the end of 1985 William Haseltine of the Harvard Medical School estimated that in New York City, one out of three prostitutes probably had AIDS, partly because so many of them either are junkies or live with junkies; and, in New York City, 59 percent of the junkies are estimated to have been exposed to AIDS.

In fact, this "muddying factor" may be contaminating not just the study of prostitutes with AIDS, but all AIDS cases, heterosexual and homosexual. Sexual activity may not have the significance in the transmission of AIDS that most researchers have assumed.

The difficulty in making any definite statement about the connection between drugs and AIDS is that recreational drug use is so widespread the high percentage of people with AIDS who have used street drugs may be only a reflection of the high percentage of people in general, with AIDS or without, who have snorted, inhaled, and swallowed powders, pot, and pills over the past couple of decades.

Even though drug use and abuse *may* be more significant than sex in giving AIDS to prostitutes, many hookers have become very cautious. One woman, a prostitute for seven years, claimed that "*all* of the call girls, streetwalkers, working cocktail waitresses, escorts, and masseuses I've known in the northern, central, and southern parts of California *use condoms religiously* for intercourse acts. . . . There are no 'safe customers.' Only in slave labor situations and legalized counties in Nevada do those supposedly 'clean' ladies expose themselves to repeated contacts [without condoms] on a daily basis." And, on East Eighty-sixth Street, one of New York's streetwalker strips, the hookers are so terrified of getting the disease that when they give blowjobs, at the last minute they pop a plastic bag in their mouths.

10.

As for women who have sex with bisexual men. . . . Researchers generally described them as "sexually active." They had, according to one study used by the New York City Department of Health, "One to 30 . . . partners, with a median of 2.5 partners." It wasn't clear what a *.5 partner* was: maybe one who just dry-humps.

Some researchers seemed to feel that disease was the natural consequence of their behavior. It wasn't that they deserved what they got; it was more a commitment to moral logic: Effect follows cause. A researcher, catching himself disapproving of how much the women in the risk group seemed to sleep around, tried to redeem himself by explaining that it wasn't a matter of quantity so much as quality. He could understand "normal" sex drives, he said; but why did they go to bed with bisexuals? In other words: If they're gonna be nymphos, they should at least save it for Real Men—presumably Alpha Males like him.

11.

Some women who are neither prostitutes nor promiscuous seem drawn to junkies and make up a risk group that has not gotten much attention.

"They're often people who have father trouble," said Joan, who during a two-and-a-half-year period lived first with one junkie and then another. "They"—she shrugged—"*we* feel an inability to fit into regular society. Junkies are just as alienated, maybe more, so in comparison we don't feel so out of it. Junkies also feed our self-pity. And we can be overwhelmingly maternal with junkies, who are like kids you have to take care of. The broken-wing syndrome."

She met her first junkie at Danceteria, a Manhattan club, where she had met a number of junkies. "This is *it,*" she thought. He was a Viet vet who claimed he got hooked during the war; but he was on drugs before he enlisted. "He could be immensely likable," she said. "The situation seemed romantic, different. I closed my eyes to a lot of the stealing he did, kept believing he was going to kick the drugs. Finally I kicked him out."

She swore never to get involved with a junkie again, but the first night she spent with the next man she ended up living with she saw needle marks on his arms. Again, she went ahead with the relationship. He also could be charming.

"Junkie number one and junkie number two," she said. "Like the things that come out of the box in *The Cat in the Hat.*"

And like the creatures from *The Cat in the Hat,* they stopped being fun, became sinister, and almost wrecked her life. Even after she stopped seeing them, broke herself of the junkie-lover habit, they still disrupted her life. When she first heard about AIDS and about how women who'd had sex with junkies were at risk, she panicked. For weeks she could think of nothing else. Every time she got a sniffle, she was convinced she had the disease.

She said, "People say, 'Don't make love to anyone you don't know really well. If you're not sure of where they've been or what they've been doing, stick to heavy petting.'

But it's different for me. I'm afraid to be with anyone now. Not because I might get it, but because I'm afraid I'll give it to some guy I care about"—sharing with them what was shared with her. Corruption is generous.

Both junkie number one and junkie number two wanted to draw Joan into their vice. In both cases the sharing of the needles was part of the allure of the drug.

"There was some communion in it," she said. "Something sexual. The insertion."

The compulsion to incorporate into the body something alien is not necessarily as bizarre as it sounds. It may stem from a healthy effort to escape solipsism, a desire to experience a reality that isn't the product of one's own consciousness, to hear the tree falling in the forest that no one is around to hear.

Or it may come from the same impulse as love, a need to find someone or something *other* that can, in some unclear and perhaps mysterious way, complete the self. Plato claimed that originally men and women were single spherical beings that broke apart, leaving each now-separate sex forever cut off from and forever craving the other, the Platonic twin. In love, such yearning to join selves—even when the desire to merge may be the emotional equivalent of shooting up—is seen as heroic, the mark of true passion, a rare state that is so pursued it lies at the heart of much of Western literature and art, feeds popular romances, television, and movies, and powers advertising.

So the same thing that makes junkies needle freaks—and makes some women junkie freaks—may make us all romantics. And may drive us all to find outside ourselves something that will make us feel complete, whether that something is healthy or unhealthy, love or drugs, or sex, or even the ultimate other, the thing most alien and that

therefore offers the most intense feeling of completion—
Death.

12.

One CDC researcher called the AIDS risk groups the
4-H Club: homos, heroine addicts, Haitians, and hookers.

AIDS wasn't a disease that hit "respectable" people. It
was almost as though the germs themselves—if the disease
was caused by germs—were layabouts, marginal microorganisms from the wrong side of the tracks. Not aristocratic
like the disorder that causes hemophilia, the bane of gen-
erations of European royalty.

Then it turned out hemophiliacs were coming down with
this Gay Plague. And patients who'd had blood transfusions, some of whom were children.

Suddenly the straight world got concerned. It wasn't just
happening to faggots, junkies, hookers, and Haitians. It was
hitting hemophiliacs and kids—even kids! The disease was
no better than a child molester. Perhaps, most frightening
of all—it was affecting people who'd had transfusions. Anyone might need a transfusion. Anyone. You. Me.

A rumor started in Texas that AIDS could be transmitted to the blood donor. In less than a week donations at one
of the largest blood banks in the country, the New York
Blood Center, dropped by 25 percent.

"What happened was a minor panic," said Dr. Alan
Waldman, a researcher at the blood center. "It was blown
completely out of proportion—to some extent by the media
and particularly by Geraldo Rivera, a New York broad-
caster, who reported [for ABC News's "20/20"] that the
nation's blood supply was in danger. The distinction was

blurred between responsible blood donation centers and off-the-street pay-for-the-pint commercial operations."

"The CDC is responsible for the panic," said Dr. Aaron Kellner, head of the New York Blood Center. "You shouldn't yell *fire* in a crowded theater—even if there is a fire—because the resulting panic can cause more deaths than the threat."

Although experts estimated the chance of blood contamination to be 1 in 100,000, people are convinced they're going to win lotteries on longer odds than that. No one wanted to give or get transfusions.

The Medical and Scientific Advisory Council of the National Hemophilia Foundation recommended a ban on accepting blood donated by people in the high-risk groups.

It might be easy to spot the junkies—at least the indigent, in ragged clothes, their arms blue and scarred, ready to sell their regular amount to a commercial outfit. But how can you tell a homosexual? Do you demand a sexual history of everyone who offers to donate blood? What about gay men who work in corporations who are expected to give blood and who are in the closet?

"We developed a confidential questionnaire that allowed them [blood donors] to check whether they wanted the blood to be used for transfusion or research," said Dr. Joanna Pyndike, head of the Greater New York Blood Program.

That solved the problem of assuring donors privacy. But the myth of the healthy donor who gets infected continued to spread. In a Roper poll of two thousand individuals, 91 percent had heard of AIDS, probably more than those who knew the name of the vice president of the United States. And 26 percent thought you could get it from giving blood.

By the fall of 1982, around the time of the blood donation crisis, the number of AIDS cases had risen to 593. Two hundred and forty-three of the people with AIDS—41 percent—had died.

One of the CDC epidemiologists said, "We had never seen this problem in nature before."

4 / Theories

We may never discover the secret of the deadliness of Spanish influenza because it was a matter of the balance between two factors, each of which defines the other, i.e., the virus' virulence and the hosts' vulnerability.

—Alfred W. Crosby, Jr.,
Epidemic and Peace, 1918

1.

AIDS is an epidemiologist's dream: A mystery disease. That is fatal. That hits specific populations. Every small-town doctor, big-city intern, academic researcher, and government grant hound wanted to try his wit against the disease. In America the major centers of AIDS research and study are the Centers for Disease Control, the National Institutes of Health, the New York Blood Center, Harvard University, New York Hospital–Cornell Medical Center, and Sloan-Kettering. Abroad the leading research center for AIDS is the Pasteur Institute in Paris. Although these organizations have a lock on most of the government grants and big-time names, many smaller research facilities, like San Francisco's Mt. Zion Hospital and Medical Center and the AIDS Medical Foundation in New York City, are also doing significant work.

Since AIDS cripples the immune system, a solution to the crisis can lead to a profound understanding of how the immune system works—how the body fights off all disease. Whoever discovered that would revolutionize medicine. The search for the cause of and cure for AIDS became a race. What was at stake might be nothing less than the Nobel Prize.

2.

Trying to figure out what caused AIDS was like playing Chutes and Ladders. As new information came in, you could make remarkably quick advances and suffer equally quick reverses. Everyone had a pet theory for AIDS. Environmental. Psychosocial. Genetic. Viral. Some people looked at defects in the host. Others looked to causes outside the host.

The best clue researchers had was the abnormalities in the immune system.

The immune system is the body's complex and still imperfectly understood defense mechanism. Its job is to tell the difference between Self and Not-Self. A splinter is Not-Self; the toe it's embedded in is Self. The bacteria that keep you home from work with aches and fever, wrapped up in a quilt and watching reruns of "My Little Margie," is Not-Self; pyrogen, the substance that may cause the rise in your temperature, is Self.

The immune system is made up of two parts: the cellular immune system, which directly attacks pathogens (Not-Self, alien invaders of the body like bacteria or viruses), and the more powerful humoral immune system, which indirectly attacks pathogens by producing antibodies. Antibodies are proteins that identify and lock on to foreign substances, tagging them so they can be recognized and destroyed by different kinds of protector cells.

A baby is born with an immature immune system, which in time develops the ability to tell Self from Non-Self, the same thing the child must do psychologically. What's

Mama, and what's me? A question that, at first, does not have a clear-cut answer either psychologically or physiologically.

In newborns some antibodies come from the mother. These maternal antibodies are temporary bodyguards, holding the line while the kid develops his or her own antibodies. The mother's antibodies for measles may last in her child's system for as long as a year. A child's immune system isn't fully mature until he or she is about eleven years old—when the antibodies found (among other places) in tears have reached adult levels—the same time kids begin rebelling against their parents, dramatizing that they are individuals. The physiological and psychological Selves achieve adult status at the same time.

A chart of how the immune system works looks like a diagram of a football play: circles with abbreviations in them, arrows pointing from one circle to another and making curves around the outside. The Home Team—the leukocytes (the white blood cells)—is divided into two groups of protector cells: the phagocytes and the lymphocytes.

A homophobic, or perhaps merely homohostile, scientist joked that phagocytes, which he sniggeringly spelled on a blackboard *fagocytes,* were cells "whose job is to kill off fags," one of many examples among male heterosexuals of a kind of social immune system, an aggressive attempt made very early in my interviews with them to distinguish Self from Not-Self. In these cases Self and Not-Self were corporate identities: straight men versus gay men.

"As a heterosexual," a scientist would say—and then launch into some technical discussion that had nothing to do with sexual orientation.

We. They. Us. Them.

Invariably the people I interviewed would subtly probe, trying to find out if I was gay without coming right out and asking. Unable to decide, they tended to be circumspect in how they discussed the disease and the risk groups. But if, halfway through the interview, I let them know I was straight, abruptly the tone of the conversation changed, became confidential; they'd betray a club man's smug assumption of shared amusement at the outlandish antics of The Others.

The scientist corrected his deliberate misspelling.

"*Phago* comes from the Greek"—he smirked, but resisted making the obvious joke—"*phagein,* which means 'to eat'; *-cyte* comes from the Greek *kytos,* which means 'cell.' Phagocytes are Self that eat Not-Self."

Again he smirked.

"Why is it," he asked, "everything I say today seems to have a double meaning?"

Phagocytes are cellular Pac-Men that roam the body looking for invaders—bacteria, for example—to destroy. They are divided into two groups: macrophages and granulocytes. And they can destroy aliens in two ways: by absorbing and digesting them (as macrophages do) or kamikazi-style by destroying themselves along with the invader (as granulocytes do).

Lymphocytes are also divided into two groups: B-cells and T-cells.

B-cells, which get their training in the bone marrow, produce the various antibodies. One kind of antibody, a cellular condiment, coats antigens like ketchup on a hamburger so macrophages will eat them. Another, like a spy's secret transmitter hidden on a bad guy, tells the phagocytes where the action is, so they can stage a raid. A third—the kind found in tears—forms a shield past which microorganisms can't go. This is the humoral immunity system.

The cellular immune system involves the T-cells, which can be divided into two major groups: T-helpers and T-suppressors. T-helper, also called T-4, cells help B-cells produce antibodies.

It is among T-helper cells that AIDS seems to wreak most havoc. The AIDS virus infects T-helper cells, subverting them and preventing them from recognizing foreign substances and from stimulating the production of B-cells, which in turn prevents the B-cells from producing the antibodies that could help destroy the AIDS viruses. Inside the infected T-helper cells, the AIDS virus multiplies. Then the new generation of AIDS viruses bursts from the infected T-helper cells, each new virus ready to infect its own T-cell. The production of AIDS viruses and infection of T-helper cells increases geometrically.

T-suppressor cells, also called T-8 cells, are leukocytic party poopers that go around frustrating the activities of the T-helpers—just so things won't get out of control. Under normal circumstances you don't want your immune system to become too aggressive. Like a democratic state put under martial law that continues long after the crisis is over, your body could put into effect emergency measures worse than what prompted them, leading to a kind of organic paranoia in which the body, convinced its own cells are betraying it, attacks and destroys them. The results? Allergic reactions. Anemia. Even certain cancers.

Usually the ratio of T-helper to T-suppressor cells is two to one. In AIDS patients it is usually reversed. In some cases the person with AIDS may have virtually no T-helper cells at all.

So not only does the AIDS virus seem to prevent T-helper cells from doing their job but, by reversing the normal ratio of T-helper cells to T-suppressor cells, the AIDS virus enlists the T-suppressors in subverting the immune system. It uses the body's natural ability to suppress the activity of the T-helper cells against itself.

Other parts of the immune system don't fit into a scheme quite so simply. One T-cell, called a killer cell, works independently to wipe out invaders. The immune system also has an assassin called the natural killer cell, which goes to work without first having to check back with T-lymphocyte Central. Unlike the T-cells, which know which antigens to attack because they've encountered them before, the natural killer cell doesn't have any previous experience with a particular invader. It's an alien; that's enough.

There are also interferons, which inhibit viruses from reproducing and stimulate growth of certain cells (like the natural killers) that can attack viruses. And interleukin-2, a hormone that helps activate T-helper cells.

So: phagocytes eat antigens; and T-helpers stimulate B-cells, which produce antibodies, which coat antigens, which induce phagocytes to eat them or stimulate the creation of a substance (called *complement*) that sets up a "Hey, Rube!" to attract phagocytes to a point of infection. T-killers and natural killers destroy antigens. T-suppressors sabotage the system—in order to save it.

The football play the diagram of the immune system looks like could have been planned by the Marx Brothers.

Invaders, defenders, front lines, skirmishes, sieges. The similes and metaphors used to describe the immune system tend to be drawn from the military. Or sports, demonology, and science fiction.

It's hard to escape the comparisons, because fear of disease dredges up childish anxieties that tend to express themselves in childish images. To escape, we want to believe that all we must do is duck under our desks with our arms crossed over our heads. Facing what we can't avoid is as excruciating as being fifth-graders scrimmaging against sixth-graders.

Possession by evil spirits. Aliens seizing our neighbors

and seductively urging us to surrender to the inevitable. When we are faced with serious—and mysterious—disease, our lives are taken over by all the props and conventions of a Saturday-afternoon matinee. *Banzai!* *"Win one for the—"* *"Your mother sucks cocks in Hell!"* *"But you've got to believe me, officer; they've landed!"*

In the light of day the nightmares fade. We leave the theaters, blinking, feeling both satisfied and foolish at having been frightened. The Japs were not World War II monsters, just enemy patriots. Football is only a game. The worst damnation Satan offers while speaking through the mouth of a possessed child is a—presumably anonymous but innocuous—sex act; the *mother* part diminishing rather than increasing the horror by making the Devil sound like nothing more terrifying than a rank-out artist.

Even though it may be helpful to use figures of speech to explain a complex function, metaphors and similes may be subliminally misleading. T-cells are not infantrymen. B-cells are not linebackers. People with AIDS are not possessed by either evil spirits or pods from another galaxy. And the immune system is not a useful model for a grade-B genre movie; it is a biological process upon which our lives depend—the process that goes awry in people with AIDS.

3.

Changes in the ratios of T-helper cells and T-suppressor cells can be monitored by using a cell sorter, an instrument for analyzing AIDS blood, which looks like a machine designed to zap life into the Golem: a laser tube filled with argon gas, mirrors, switches, meters, filters, metal plates with 6,000 volts crackling between them—everything but bubbling green liquids and lightning rods to attract zigzag bolts. At the New York Blood Center, one of the country's largest blood bank and blood research laboratories, the cell sorter takes up two rooms, one for the computer that analyzes the cells and another for the machine you feed the cells through.

"Say I've got some blood," said Dr. Jay Valinsky, the assistant director of the Greater New York Blood Program at the New York Blood Center, an intense, enthusiastic man who gives the impression of being as good-hearted and absentminded as Fred MacMurray in *The Son of Flubber,* the kind of guy who might dreamily put his coffee cup under a dripping retort and sip from a test tube. On the wall right outside the cell sorter room was a movie poster of Dracula, an appropriate decoration for a blood bank. "And say I want to look at T-helper/T-suppressor ratios. Here's a pot of cells that I've stained with antihelper antibody [fluorescent markers that attach themselves to T-helper cells]. Here's a pot of cells that I've stained with antisuppressor antibody [fluorescent markers that will attach themselves to T-suppressor cells]."

He put the liquid into the machine, which forced it through some spaghetti tubing and out a nozzle made from a sapphire with a tiny hole drilled in it. The hole is so small, the jet of liquid that spurts out has cells lined up single file. One by one the cells drip through a laser, which shimmered with an eerie light as grainy as a half-tone photograph in a newspaper.

"Don't put your finger in the beam," Valinsky said. "Half the power of this laser could easily burn a hole in a piece of paper.

"When the laser light hits one of the cells, two things happen," Valinsky said. First, the light scatters—just as if you shot a handful of Ping-Pong balls at a basketball. The Ping-Pong balls would bounce back. The larger the target—say, a beach ball instead of a basketball—the more Ping-Pong balls would hit and ricochet. The bigger the cell, the more light gets scattered. This measures the size of the cell dropping past the laser light.

Second, the laser light excites the fluorescent antibody bound to the cell. The more antibody molecules attached to the cell, the more intense the fluorescence; the intensity of the fluorescence identifies what kind of cell it is, a T-helper or not; a T-suppressor cell or not.

You can also count how many cells have passed through the laser beam. And you can sort the cells, separate them—make T-helpers drip into one test tube and T-suppressors drip into another test tube.

"Here's what happens," said Valinsky. "Here's the stream. The cells are lined up. . . ." The laser hits a cell. The light scatters, and the cell fluoresces. The information zips over to the computer and gets analyzed. The cell continues dropping past the laser. The analyzed information zips back and gives the cell (say, a T-helper cell) a positive charge. (As they drip, other cells, which are not T-helper cells, will get negatively charged.) The stream of liquid is vibrated forty thousand times a second to break it up into droplets, one cell in each droplet. The T-helper cell, now charged, continues dropping. It passes between two deflection plates, which have also been electrically charged and act like magnets, the positive plate attracting the negatively charged cells and making them swerve in one direction and fall into a test tube on that side of the machine, the negatively charged plate attracting the positively charged cells and making them swerve in the other direction and fall into a test tube on the other side of the machine. The positively charged T-helper cell swings toward the negative deflector plate and drips into the T-helper cell test tube.

"We have to hit the cell with the laser," Valinsky said,

"get the information, analyze it, and send it back with a charge in something less than a hundred microseconds."

I peered through a lens at the droplets breaking off from the stream and falling one by one. A strobe light made it look as if the droplets were not moving.

An ink jet graphs the information, a dot for each cell, on paper. Little and dim cells get dots in the lower left quadrant. Big and bright cells get dots in the upper right quadrant.

"One could do this with a microscope," Valinsky said. "But that's a very subjective job. If you want to score whether a cell is positive or negative"—how fluorescent it is—"you sometimes have to look at it for a long time before making a decision. Here the machine does it for you—precisely. It will resolve much smaller differences because the eye is just not as sensitive."

He checked a readout.

"Doing it by microscope also takes a longer time," he said. "While we were talking, I just collected thirteen thousand cells. How long did it take us to do this? Fifteen seconds. With a microscope, to count thirteen thousand cells would probably take me six years."

The cell sorter and the technique of tagging T-helper and T-suppressor cells with fluorescent markers have both come into common use in only the past half-dozen years.

"Since 1975–76," Valinsky said.

Just a few years before AIDS was recognized. About the same time doctors began routinely carrying out the operation that allows them to confirm a diagnosis of pneumocystis.

"Everything happened simultaneously," Valinsky said.

"It's possible," said one of Valinsky's colleagues, "people were dying of AIDS ten years ago, but we just didn't know it was AIDS then."

According to a report in *Science News* the AIDS virus may have been in blood frozen in 1972.

Valinsky led me through the blood center   the preparation lab for the cell sorter with its centrifuge, hallways that had the sulfurous smell of hypo in a photography darkroom and that were crowded with liquid nitrogen tanks in which frozen cells were stored, rooms in which cells were grown in incubators labeled Nursery 1, Nursery 2, and Bordello.

"If you're doing a short-term experiment," Valinsky said, "quick in and out, you use the bordello."

At the autoclave, a pressurized steam sterilizer that looks like a large, elongated clothes dryer, Valinsky talked about laboratory decontamination, a subject that became important as soon as there was the possibility that AIDS might be caused by an infectious agent. In November of 1982 the CDC published guidelines for clinical and laboratory staffs that said even though "Airborne spread and interpersonal spread through casual contact do not seem likely," it "appears prudent for hospital personnel to use the same precautions . . . as those used for patients with hepatitis B virus infection, in which blood and body fluids likely to have been contaminated with blood are considered infective."

A list of doctors' do's and don'ts, many of them common sense, followed. Don't stick yourself with a needle used on an AIDS patient; wear gloves "when handling blood specimens, blood-soaked items, body fluids, excretions, and secretions, as well as surfaces, materials, and objects exposed to them"; wear gowns, too; wash hands after removing gloves; make sure you clearly label AIDS specimens; and clean up blood spills "promptly."

Some of the rules for researchers were the same as those for physicians, but there were a few new ones, like: Don't suck AIDS blood or fluids into pipettes with your mouth (use "mechanical pipetting devices"). And: Try to keep

AIDS-contaminated blood and body fluids from spraying around the labs.

"What we generally do is put all the solutions that have ever come in contact with a potentially harmful agent into Clorox [bleach], which is a very strong oxydizing agent," Valinsky said. "That usually kills the virus."

Usually?

They also flush out the spaghetti tubing and other parts of the machine with Clorox. All potentially AIDS-laced liquids end up "in that plastic jug sitting down there, which also has Clorox in it," Valinsky said.

What happens to that?

"That gets dumped."

"Where?"

"Down the toilet."

"There's no danger?"

"To be honest," Valinsky said, "I don't know."

They also pump any AIDS-contaminated mist "up through this tube and to this filter system and out into the air," Valinsky said. "It's filtered with filters with very small pores in it. It will filter bacteria."

And viruses?

"It won't filter viruses."

What if AIDS is a virus?

"They're the same kind of filters used in the hepatitis lab upstairs," he said.

When I asked Dr. David Sencer, then head of New York City's Department of Health, about the decontamination procedures, he blinked rapidly a few times while his press aide frantically scribbled a note on a yellow pad and, hiding the words from me, held it up like a cue card for him to read.

I asked Valinsky if he uses a mask when he works with AIDS blood.

He shook his head no.

"But nobody has gotten anything?" I asked.

"Well," he said, "we've been working with the stuff for a year and a half."

The assumed incubation time for AIDS might be up to two or three or even five years.

"Doesn't it make you nervous?" I asked.

"Yup," he said, adding, presumably to explain how he handled his nervousness, "I hate to say it, but often I feel that if you can't see it, it can't hurt you."

It's possible that the virus is so vulnerable it can be killed by simple detergent, or even soap and water.

He continued: "We like people to wear gloves when they're handling the samples. We encourage the people who are using gloves to take them off before they go around touching door handles. We reviewed it all with the New York Department of Health a year ago. We all pretty much agree this is the best we can do right now. As I say, *If it works out, great!*"

"And if it doesn't?" I asked.

Down the sink. Out into New York's air.

He grinned. "There's not much we can do about it."

4.

So researchers count and sort T-cells and find the abnormal ratios. Still, the T-cell ratios are only the shadow cast by the disease. The question remained: What's causing the abnormalities? The environment? Genetics? A virus?

Environment includes all external agents: from poppers to mysterious toxic substances unique to the areas where there was a concentration of people who came down with

AIDS. DDT, for example, is a powerful immunosuppressor. So is radiation.

"If you look at dioxin," said Dr. Celso Bianco, the director of the Greater New York Blood Program Laboratory, whose office was down the hall from Valinsky's, "whoof! It is a most powerful immunosuppressive agent."

Bianco, hands folded behind his head, gazed at the ceiling as though he were settling back in a planetarium, ready for a star show. He was a short, pudgy man with the subversive wit of a radical priest—like the hero of *The Little World of Don Camillo* or a character in a Vittorio De Sica movie. He was the colleague of Valinsky's who'd suggested that maybe what was new was not AIDS but the technology to identify it—and the conditions that may have caused an eruption of the disease in the middle class.

"I don't think there's a convincing theory," he said. "Every theory has a hole. For any theory I could be either the prosecutor or the defense attorney."

A thorough scientist, he gave every possibility its day in court.

Maybe AIDS developed out of conditions (like chemical wastes) similar to those poisoning the Love Canal—although in discussing that theory one runs the danger of linguistic confusion. A researcher had a long and puzzling conversation with a gay man who had never heard of the hazardous wastes landfill near Niagara Falls; it took them nearly half an hour to realize that the gay guy thought the scientist was using "love canal" as a euphemism.

But the poisons that can suppress the immune system aren't necessarily concentrated in toxic dumps. Humankind has polluted the planet with all sorts of immunosuppressors. Three years before the first CDC report on AIDS, Dr. Bianco wrote in an essay, "Resisting Pollution": "Despite their extraordinary arsenals, our bodies seem ill-prepared for the twentieth century. They have difficulty fending off assaults from the legacy of the industrial revolution: smoke, radiation, food additives, polluted water, and industrial chemicals such as asbestos and vinyl chloride." The poisons we have spewed into our environment have helped lower our resistance to many diseases, not just AIDS. Just like the poisons we take for recreation.

A National Institutes of Health study, done in conjunction with the Navy and the Uniformed Services Medical School, suggested that amyl nitrite use could suppress the immune system, which might leave someone vulnerable to a virus (if AIDS were a virus) or lead directly to the opportunistic infections and Kaposi's. On the other hand, the CDC (which has a competitive relationship with the National Institutes of Health that no one wants to admit) found no convincing link between amyl and AIDS.

My cat just dropped a shrew beside my desk. Shrews are one of nature's nastiest beasts, sort of criminal moles. Night creatures with sharp reddish-tipped teeth, poisonous saliva, and so high strung—their evil hearts beat 1,200 times a minute—they hardly ever sleep and spend most of their waking hours feeding with a terrifying ferocity. Imagine a four-inch shark disguised as a mouse.

On my bookshelf I happened to have the other bottle of butyl nitrite I'd bought in Los Angeles—which, out of a curiosity somewhat less scientific than that which motivated the researchers who gave amyl to rats, I opened and held toward the shrew. The animal did the *Insectivora* equivalent of a Marty Feldman imitation.

Although by the end of 1982 most people had crossed poppers off the list of causes, there is renewed speculation that poppers may be somehow connected to AIDS. Researchers at the National Jewish Center for Immunology and Respiratory Medicine have found that butyl nitrite seems linked to increased risk of an AIDS-like disease in mice.

Steroid creams, which are used on herpes sores and hemorrhoids and which have an immunosuppressive effect, had a brief boom among researchers. But there wasn't any significant correlation between the medication and people with AIDS, so that theory quickly faded.

At first there seemed to be a good chance there was a genetic link to AIDS. Genetics might explain the Haitian connection. And there was the tendency of Kaposi's to hit Jews and Italians. Eighty percent of the AIDS patients with Kaposi's shared a genetic marker called the HLA-DR5 (a group of genes with a particular component). But over time the percentage of Kaposi's patients with that genetic marker dropped from 80 percent to 43 percent. It's possible the high percentage that showed up at first was simply due to a sociological quirk, something as humdrum as the similarity (at least in myth) between Jewish and Italian mothers, who (also according to myth) behave in ways that might cause a greater proportion of their sons to become homosexual; or a geographical quirk, something as obvious as the high proportion of Jews and Italians in New York City, which had the highest number of AIDS cases.

Or maybe some homosexuality was genetic—a view entertained by panelists at the 1985 annual convention of the American Psychological Association—and AIDS was a characteristic linked to a specific biological makeup, which would explain why some gays got it while their roommates did not. Perhaps someone picks up the agent by "behaving in unusual ways"—sniffing poppers or wallowing in a backroom—but the agent needs particular conditions, genetic or otherwise, in order to take hold.

Still, even if environment and genetics were co-factors,

states that led to AIDS susceptibility, apparently neither was the prime cause of the disease. Or diseases.

"Remember," Bianco said, "AIDS is a name we give to a number of different conditions. It is a breakdown of the immune system, and I can think of two or three dozen places where the breakdown could occur. It is possible we are mixing in the same bag a lot of different things."

5.

Every mystery has a center of gravity that keeps tugging the detective, a central point to which he or she must return, the drag of reality. In a murder mystery it is identity of the victim. Who was killed can explain why the murder took place. In a medical mystery it is the identity of the patient. Who got sick? The best detective is the one who pays closest attention to the obvious.

From the very beginning most of the people wtih AIDS were gay. (After a preliminary shakedown, the proportion of gay AIDS patients has remained fairly constant: roughly 75 percent.)

Why so many gays? And why has the proportion of gays with AIDS remained so constant?

Since the key didn't seem to be what gays were, Dr. Steve Witkin at the Cornell Medical Center in New York City decided to look at what gays did. Not what drugs they took, not what places they went to, but something in their sexual practices that might make them more susceptible than straights.

Witkin said, "I personally believe that the average person"—by which he apparently meant male heterosexuals who are neither junkies, Haitians, hemophiliacs, nor people in need of transfusions—"is not at risk for AIDS."

What's the difference between the "average person" and a male homosexual?

Semen.

Witkin is so sure his theory is right and that there is no danger to straights that he regularly eats his lunch in his laboratory—which has a sign on the door: *Biohazard: AIDS biological material.* In the hall outside is a safety shower, so if you get contaminated you can immediately wash yourself off. Beside his desk was a note—like the kind that used to be left on the back porch for the milkman—reminding Witkin, "AIDS sera in refrigerator every Tuesday."

Witkin had the same combination of innocence and knowingness found in an eighteenth-century cherub, like one of the sly cupids fussing with Venus's hair in a Boucher painting. He seemed guileless, oblivious to medical politics.

On the wall of his laboratory were messages and pictures from his children. *I love my dad. He fights diseases. I love my dad. He's the best scientist in the world.* Once, when his eight-year-old daughter, Jolene, visited the lab, she typed:

The AIDS

The AIDS is a very bad disease. . . . People that have the AIDS can die. The AIDS is very bad. If you have the AIDS, please contact Cornell Medical Center.

Witkin didn't have any hidden agenda, any bias to defend; he wasn't on a moral crusade. He seemed motivated simply by the desire to save lives, which is what made his research—or the implications of his research—so disturbing.

Since so many "sexually active" gays got AIDS, Witkin and his colleagues reasoned, it seemed logical to conclude that "the syndrome may have some relation to circulating antibodies evoked as a result of semen deposition in the alimentary canal." In other words, someone else's semen, shot up your ass, might cause your body to produce antibodies to the foreign semen, which in turn could suppress the immune system, leaving it unable to fight off infection by the AIDS-associated diseases or by an AIDS virus that might itself further damage the immune system.

To test this semen–immune system theory, Witkin explained, "We took rabbits and gave them rabbit semen rectally once a week." Not enormous amounts; "a small dose," Witkin said, something comparable to what a "sexually active" gay man might get. "Healthy males [rabbits] were restrained and 1 ml of fresh semen . . . was deposited . . . to a depth of 5 cm . . . with a No. 7 French rubber catheter."

The scientific method is alien to the world of the sexual underground, gay or straight—the peep shows and live sex shows, the gay baths and strip joints, the world of prostitutes and fast-track anonymous encounters; S-M, B-D, the whole alphabet of perverse desire. The two worlds—one rational and the other impulsive, repel each other like similar poles of two magnets. They don't connect. The gap between can be bridged only by absurdity. A scientific freak show. Or Looney-Toons laboratories.

I had visions of bunny bondage: Harvey, the White Rabbit from *Alice in Wonderland*, Peter Rabbit, Peter Cottontail, the Easter Bunny, and Bugs all strapped down in brass beds; Uncle Wiggily, a red bandanna replacing the white handkerchief that usually stuck out of his back right pocket, lurking into a shop on Forty-second Street to buy a set of butt plugs; the Hare from the Aesop story letting the Tortoise win because he stopped to cruise some jackrabbits; the cuddly hero of *Pat the Bunny* being buggered with a No. 7 French catheter—whatever that was—so gently its rectum was not traumatized.

An earlier study had found that when semen is injected

intravenously into rats, antisperm antibody is produced. Witkin wanted to make sure it was the introduction of semen, not the trauma—or the semen entering the bloodstream through abrasions or cuts—that affected the immune system.

Saltwater was squirted up the asses of a group of control rabbits.

"How did you get the rabbit semen?" I asked.

Witkin looked surprised that I didn't know the obvious answer.

"Just use an artificial [rabbit] vagina," he said.

The rabbits, both those buggered and those from which Witkin got the semen, were originally healthy. Just as he had suspected, "In six to eight weeks, the rabbits [who were getting the semen] developed antibodies to the sperm, antibodies that reacted with the immune system."

The rabbits getting saltwater did not develop antibody to sperm.

So, I asked, is semen dangerous? (I had a flash of a future that mimicked the past: All sex reduced to the customs of 1959, women shrinking from going all the way—because it involved sperm—and men promising to pull out before ejaculation. *Just let me put the tip in, just the tip, just for a second!* The hand jive of hand jobs. A bull market in condoms— which, in fact, has happened: Women, who used to make up a negligible part of the market, now account for 40 percent of all condom sales.)

But, Witkin explained, sperm was not dangerous when introduced vaginally.

"The cells lining the vagina are different from the cells in the rectum," he said.

So heterosexual fucking was safe.

And sperm was not dangerous when introduced orally, Witkin went on.

So blowjobs—heterosexual or homosexual—were safe.

But, I assumed, anal sex, whether heterosexual or homosexual, was not.

Not necessarily, Witkin said.

Although there was one study done in Texas and reported in *The Journal of the American Medical Association* that suggested that women who have anal sex might respond in a similar way to men who have anal sex, developing antisperm antibody and having their immune system suppressed, that was not conclusive. Witkin thought women were not at risk even if they had anal sex—or rather even if their partners ejaculated inside them during anal intercourse.

And this was the troubling part of the interview.

"Females," Witkin said, "have evolved immunological mechanisms to deal with exposure to sperm."

They had to in order for the species to continue.

But men did not have to evolve immunological mechanisms to deal with exposure to sperm.

The implication was that gay sex—at least gay anal sex—is biologically unnatural.

I suppose this was the point at which my true feelings about gay sex were tested. I had tentative scientific support for bigotry. If I wanted an excuse to dismiss homosexuality, I could use Witkin's experiment.

It's true I have little patience with stereotypes: both those that bigots believe in and those indulged in by people who are ready to surrender their individuality. The biker, the banker, the hard-hat, the swish—I distrust anyone, gay or straight, who accepts a set of received ideas, whether they are corporate, political, cultural, or sexual. I dislike clones—and I don't mean the word in just the gay sense. Heterosexuals mimic fashion and imitate behavior that is presented as desirable as much as homosexuals do.

Such a surrender to style is reductive (in how it simplifies, in how it eliminates options) and totalitarian (not in the political sense but in its effect on individual choice). But I recognize that anyone who gives in to a particular fashion may be merely seeking to reintroduce ritual into a life stripped of ceremony. Ritual repeats; it has no surprises. A priest doesn't improvise in a mass; a rabbi doesn't rewrite the *sh'ma*. A clone of any kind follows a particular style, in dress or speech or manners, to renew his or her kinship with others. It is a tribal impulse, an escape from anarchy, which is ritual's ultimate opposite.

But if there was an aspect of gay culture—or at least of the gay culture visible to the straight world—that irked me (and there was), it had less to do with homosexuality (that is, less to do with sex) than it did with class. It was what irked me about the military and the church—both of which, like gay culture, have been traditionally used by the working class as a way of rising quickly into the upper middle class. You pay for power with your freedom. It's a theme right out of a nineteenth-century novel. The kid from the provinces comes to the big city and joins the musketeers, vows allegiance to the sinister cardinal, or attaches himself to a rich homosexual in society—and suddenly is whirling in a world of luxury and adventure that would be far beyond his reach if he had stayed on the farm or apprenticed himself to the honest blacksmith in his native village.

As for gay sex, oral or anal, if I condemned it as unnatural because there may be an evolutionary bias against it, I would also have to condemn any sex act—heterosexual or homosexual or autoerotic—that did not lead to procreation.

Even more. To be consistent I would have to condemn any behavior that was not evolutionarily beneficial (that is, any behavior that threatened the continuation of a particular gene pool either because it did not lead to procreation or because it threatened the health of the procreator)—from eating hot fudge sundaes (clearly something that is not good for you: all that sugar) to flying in airplanes, from drinking Jack Daniel's to having an X-ray at the dentist's. You can make up your own list.

This is an extreme position, one that most people would properly dismiss as absurd.

Witkin's findings can easily be defended against misuse. After all, sex is friction leading to pleasure. What adults want to rub against in privacy is their own business. And people, gay or not, who follow their sexual impulses to the extreme limit of what is possible *for them* are on an odyssey as heroic—and as interesting—as Ulysses's. It takes courage to risk listening to the sirens' song.

As with all quests, most of those who sally forth end up failing, destroyed, or losing nerve; the initial enthusiasm is replaced by the grim daily struggle to survive in alien places.

When you descend into the underworld—either through the obvious entrances like New York's Hellfire Club and the rough-trade gay bars or through more subtle, disguised entrances—you must face the possibility that you may never return; not because Hell detains you by force—anyone can leave Hell anytime he wants—but because Hell offers the constant promise of fulfilling your appetite (whether the appetite is for sex, food, drugs, or knowledge) if you stay just a little longer. . . . One more orgasm will finally satisfy you. One more drink. One more snort. One more step into the unknown. One more kink. Just stay a little longer; then, you will finally be sated; then, everything will be revealed. Just stay a little longer. . . .

I suspect that a lot of the people who went to the baths

were searching not for Hell but for Paradise, an Edenic retreat in which they could indulge in sexual behavior that
was not corrupt but virtuous. By means of sexual excess
they were trying to break through to innocence—reach a
condition in which all acts were sinless because the world
was free of sin.

5 / Two Visions

The fear of disease is a happy restraint to
men. If men were more healthy, 'tis a great
chance they would be less righteous.

—A sermon preached at St. Andrew's Church,
   Holborn, England, on July 2, 1722,
   by Edmund Massey

1.

FROM the very beginning the search for the cure for AIDS was complicated by the collision of different worlds: straight versus gay, scientific versus hedonistic. There was also a clash between single-agent theories and multifactorial ones—which has been (as René Dubos pointed out in his book *Man Adapting*) a constant theme in the history of medicine. The disagreement was rooted in something more than differing analyses of statistics; it was a conflict at the heart of AIDS research, dividing the researchers into two camps, each of which has a particular vision not just of AIDS but of reality.

Those who believed AIDS was caused by a single virus (including most of the researchers at the CDC, NIH, and Harvard) betrayed a mind that was, at its extreme, amoral. The virus hits you like a bolt from the blue. What you did has nothing to do with it.

Those who believed AIDS was caused by a number of interrelated factors (like Dr. Steven Witkin at the Cornell Medical Center) betrayed a mind that was at its extreme moralistic. The disease is a direct result of how you were living your life: going to the baths, being sexually promiscuous. . . .

What each researcher looked at in his or her search for the cause of AIDS was a reflection of his or her understanding of the world. AIDS research, like any scientific study—like any attempt to describe and understand reality—was a figure-ground problem like the old chestnut from introductory psychology classes: the vase defined by the profiles of two women. When you looked at it, did you see the vase or did you see the two profiles?

The argument among AIDS researchers, it was becoming clear, was not medical as much as ontological: an argument between two world views.

Whatever it was that made someone susceptible to the disease—environment, drugs, genetics, or sperm—the disease itself, it seemed, had to be produced by an infectious agent, something similar to hepatitis B, which, because it hit the same risk groups, became a model for AIDS.

But, if AIDS—like hepatitis B—is a virus, is it an old or a new one? If it is a known virus, why is it suddenly making so many people sick? If it's a new virus, where did it come from and how did it get here? If it's a mutation, what is it a mutation of?

Of the known viruses, two candidates stood out as likely: Epstein-Barr virus (EBV) and cytomegaloviruses (CMV).

EBV depresses the immune system, has been linked to some cancers, and is associated with lymphadenopathy (which might be a pre-AIDS condition). If someone becomes immune suppressed—because of using a drug or going to too many orgies—EBV, already present in the system, clicks into gear, stimulating the B-cells, which, because the T-cells have been damaged by the immune suppression, run amok like Keystone Kops, trying to protect the body but raising havoc instead.

That was one theory.

But the epidemiological pattern didn't fit well. Everyone with AIDS did not have EBV.

The case for CMV was a little stronger.

"To follow up on the possibility of CMV being a contributing cause of AIDS, we recognized that if we just take people who already have AIDS and we culture them and look at their antibody, they're going to have CMV in their tissues or secretions or urine or semen," said Dr. Lawrence Drew. "That wouldn't tell us what we needed to know."

Drew was the director of Clinical Microbiology and the Virology Laboratory at Mt. Zion Hospital in San Francisco, California, and an associate clinical professor at the University of California (San Francisco) School of Medicine.

He had a flat face and squashed nose that made it look as if he were pressed up against a glass wall, trying to see what was on the other side. A face that looked like Buzz Sawyer's sidekick Sweeney.

Because looking for CMV antibody in people who already had AIDS would lead to self-fulfilling results, Drew and his associates decided to "find a hundred gay men who had not yet acquired CMV," Drew said. Every month they intended to check them. If their T-cell ratios became abnormal at the same time they developed CMV and if these men then came down with AIDS, the case for CMV as an agent of AIDS would look pretty good.

The facts, Drew said, support his theory. "If someone has not been infected by the virus, he has a perfectly normal helper-suppressor ratio." And if someone has been infected with CMV, "you see the very same degree of helper-suppressor abnormality that is observed in pre-AIDS and AIDS."

Since the incubation period of AIDS can be as long as

three to five years, it will take a while before Drew can see if the men who have been infected with CMV and have developed the kind of T-cell abnormalities that appear in AIDS end up getting AIDS. If they do and if CMV is one of the factors in causing AIDS, the question is why is it causing AIDS now.

"CMV has been around forever," Drew said, "so how could it be the cause? That's a little more difficult to understand, but I don't think it's impossible. With the advent of the bathhouse life-style, you had a change in the environment of the organisms. They were able to transmit much more readily than in the past. You need only look at what's going on in the so-called gay bowel syndrome. We've always had shigella and giardia, for example, but for whatever reason that was not a problem until about ten years ago" with the advent of the bathhouses.

But if CMV is being transmitted in bathhouses with an ease and intensity previously unheard of, why isn't it following its normal pattern: Someone gets it; the body fights back; and health returns. Why is it producing AIDS?

"Probably," Drew says, "because of repeated infection. If you are seeing semen in whatever orifice, you are being exposed to that virus repeatedly. The first strain may cause the [T-cell] abnormality; and, as you are recovering, you get hit with the second strain; then, the third strain."

In this theory the sperm does double duty: depressing the immune system and infecting the body with the virus.

"If you are rectally receptive," Drew said, "you have bleeding points" where the lining has been torn. If you look at the rectum through a sygmatoscope, "it looks," Drew said, "like a World War II mine field."

So having CMV-contaminated sperm shot into your ass is almost like being injected with the disease.

Since CMV can cause severe illness, whether or not it is the cause of AIDS, Drew stressed the need for prevention—at least using condoms, which he admitted help a little but aren't foolproof.

Under his direction a college student named Steve Katz Nelson did a study of how frequently condoms tend to break. In the laboratory he built a machine that mimicked sexual intercourse.

"But," Drew said, "we had to decide how many plunges" were involved in the typical fuck. They found a scientist in Seattle who in a telephone survey "had found that the average number was—I don't remember exactly, let's say fifty thrusts."

When the Seattle scientist presented his findings at a meeting, a young woman in the audience raised her hand and said, "I don't know about Seattle, but in Los Angeles it's two hundred."

Although using a condom would be advisable, the best precaution, Drew said, was not getting fucked in the ass.

From Drew's studies, male anal intercourse was the only sexual practice that correlated with CMV. The correlation was negative: men who didn't have anal intercourse had a significantly lower proportion of CMV antibody than men who did—74 percent compared to 97 percent.

"This accounts for one question," Drew said. "Why don't [more] prostitutes get AIDS?"

They're sexually active. But, Drew said, "Heterosexual men don't have the [CMV] virus in their semen to begin with. And it is predominantly heterosexual men who go to prostitutes. And, while rectal intercourse occurs in those circumstances, it isn't quite as prevalent."

According to Drew's theory, another reason relatively few women, hookers or not, get AIDS is that even if a man does have the virus in his semen, "some vaginal immunologic function" in vaginal intercourse "may help in not permitting the [CMV] virus to take root."

Also, if a man with the virus in his semen were having vaginal intercourse, it is harder for the virus to enter the bloodstream directly because the vagina's natural lubrication tends to prevent ruptures.

Despite the evidence that AIDS might be related to CMV, Drew was cautious about drawing a direct connection. If AIDS is caused by a single virus, Drew wondered, why hasn't it spread sexually in the nongay population with as much rapidity as it has been spreading in the gay population?

"If it's a one-organism/one-disease situation, there's been plenty of opportunity," he said. "There's been plenty of bisexual activity. But it isn't happening."

Even though AIDS is not spreading as rapidly in the straight population as it is in the gay population, other scientists believe that this is the result of chance—which group got the disease first. Some suspect the disease can be spread not just through anal intercourse, but through other intimate acts.

But the conclusions arrived at by Drew and his colleagues were tentatively confirmed in August of 1985. Researchers at the Pasteur Institute, the Hospital Claude Bernard, and the Université Pierre et Marie Curie in Paris and at the National Cancer Institute in the United States found evidence that in some cases CMV, EBV, and hepatitis B virus—which in another study was found to be a factor in 95 percent of the AIDS cases—may play a role in AIDS by suppressing the immune system or somehow triggering an AIDS virus.

I asked about the Haitians.

"If it were one bug," Drew said, "it would travel across the island" to the Dominican Republic.

I asked about Zaire, where there's an epidemic of what seems to be AIDS, divided roughly between men and women.

"There's only one needle in Zaire," Drew said.

I was puzzled.

Medical humor. Doctors in Zaire have to reuse needles when they are inoculating people, Drew explained. Sloppy sterilization techniques could spread the disease.

Also, according to some experts, the risk of getting AIDS may be increased by something as simple as the tendency of people to walk barefoot in certain areas in Africa: Someone with AIDS cuts his foot and leaves a spot of infected blood, which someone without AIDS who also has a cut foot steps into.

"Kids?" I asked.

Babies born with AIDS have presumably been infected in utero by their mothers, who picked up the disease through dirty needles. Other kids, who, Drew said, "came from very low socioeconomic groups," may have picked it up through filthy environments. "CMV antibody is common, because of [poor] hygiene in day-care centers, [where] it spreads quickly through urine."

"What about the case of the old couple in Florida?" I asked.

"I have trouble understanding that," Drew admitted.

Old folks can be as incontinent as infants. Maybe they picked it up in the rec room of a golden age center? Maybe they picked up CMV through contact with an infected Haitian or gay orderly. Age may have suppressed their immune systems. The answer might have been obvious if the researchers knew which questions to ask.

It turned out that the husband was a hemophiliac who got the disease through blood products and gave it to his wife during intercourse. Both were in their seventies.

Figuring out what causes AIDS is made more difficult by researcher ignorance of the subcultures that are affected by it: the elderly as well as gays and junkies. Young, healthy, white, heterosexual, nonaddicted, upper middle class, predominantly male researchers don't necessarily know what goes on in an octogenarian's bedroom, let alone what goes on in a gay bathhouse.

It would make sense for teams researching AIDS to hire someone who knew, say, both epidemiology and the gay bathhouse scene; but typically that has not been the case. Not long ago, when one gay man was hired by the CDC, he was assigned not to the AIDS Task Force, for which he was qualified and where he wanted to work, but to another division.

"I was called one time by someone who said, 'Could you tell me whether water sports are dangerous?' " Drew said. "I have kids who are extremely competitive swimmers. And I sail." On his office wall was a photograph of a boat. "I started to give some sort of answer based on swimming and sailing when he said, 'Wait a minute, here. I think we're on a different track.' "

2.

If the multifactorial theory had a champion—a knight chosen above others to do battle with the opposition—it was Dr. Joseph Sonnebend, one of the discoverers of interferon and a founder of the AIDS Medical Foundation, an independent research coordinating group. The organizations listed among members of its National Council Woody

Allen, Leonard Bernstein, Rosalyn Carter, the Reverend Theodore Hesburgh, Alan King, Paul Newman, Dr. Jonas Salk, and Jack Valenti.

Sonnebend had been treating AIDS patients since the beginning of the epidemic. When Sonnebend's activities as a doctor of AIDS patients and as an AIDS researcher became well known, the tenants in his apartment building, terrified that he would infect them all, successfully moved to have him evicted.

Sonnebend started a journal, *AIDS Research,* to publish scientific papers he believed had been excluded from mainstream scientific magazines because they explored the unpopular possibility that AIDS was a multifactorial disease.

He had a gray beard and sunken, haunted eyes. His face was haggard. He looked like a wood carving of a biblical prophet. But his manner was mild; he didn't seem ready to call God's wrath down on anyone.

He is a South African, trained in England, not part of any American old-boy network; this may explain part of his difficulty with what some feel is an AIDS mafia, a closely knit alliance of doctors and researchers who, despite their own in-fighting, have joined forces to stonewall any theory other than the single virus. Depending on whom you talk to, this mafia has its headquarters at the NIH or the CDC.

"The CDC has become the gestapo of AIDS," said one New York City health official when, out of frustration in dealing with local and federal bureaucracies, he made the decision to quit his job.

Everybody complains about everyone else. Everybody—especially in the New York gay community—distrusts everyone else.

"If I have learned one lesson from my involvement in New York gay politics, it is this," said one controversial gay leader: *"If you don't toe the party line, you don't get invited to the party."*

In a crisis, everyone has a bogeyman. The NIH has an unfair inside line on government support. The CDC blows into cities, does secret research, and vanishes back to Atlanta—without working with the local gay community. New York's Gay Men's Health Crisis Uncle Toms to the city government.

Because he has been outspoken about his beliefs, Sonnebend has drawn fire from nearly everyone, from scientists on the NIH-CDC axis to some leaders of the New York–based Gay Men's Health Crisis, which a couple of years ago ordered one of their "buddies"—one of their volunteer AIDS companions—to stop working with a nongay AIDS patient, a junkie, whom Sonnebend was trying to get into a drug detox or methadone program. Gay Men's Health Crisis had recently made it their policy not to work with junkies who were not in a detox program. The only program that would take the patient was one that demanded he be at its offices—on the Upper West Side—at seven every morning. The patient, who was quite sick, lived over an hour away, on Staten Island. Obviously the man couldn't make it. Sonnebend was trying to find a program closer to the man's home.

"I saw no reason to put him through the horrors of withdrawal while trying to get him into a program," Sonnebend said. So he continued to prescribe demerol, which the hospital had given the man.

But the "buddy" working with the man refused to drop the case and instead quit Gay Men's Health Crisis.

Sonnebend was outraged at what he thought was the Gay Men's Health Crisis's heartlessness. And he was not shy about telling people his feelings—which, of course, antagonized those who supported the Gay Men's Health Cri-

sis position. Not long after this flap, someone accused Sonnebend of irresponsibly prescribing narcotics, which, Sonnebend said, "is ridiculous. All you have to do is look at my
record" to know how carefully he prescribes drugs.

As one of the co-founders of People With AIDS–New
York, the short-lived alternative to New York Gay Men's
Health Crisis, wrote in a recent letter, "Of us all, he [Son-
nebend] has taken the most shots to the head."

3.

The offices of the AIDS Medical Foundation, near
Grand Central Station, had the provisional feel of a political campaign office: the clatter of typewriters, boxes of en-
velopes to be stuffed, the constant ringing of telephones. . . .
Sonnebend was intently giving advice to a gay man who,
afraid he had AIDS, had called in hysteria.

"If I examine you," Sonnebend said, "I'll feel better
about it."

Although he was obviously overworked and harried,
Sonnebend was offering to take on another patient. During
my interviews with him he was frequently interrupted by
the telephone to deal with someone who was sick or afraid
he was sick, and he always managed to find time for the
caller.

"You have to help," he said. "And you can't help. If
you've seen an AIDS patient in the last stages— It's one of
the most horrible ways to die. Clinicians who have been
raised in the tradition of helping can't take the helplessness.
They beat their heads against the wall. For someone who
has been taught to cure, it is a terrible, emotional thing."

He wore a gray cardigan that almost reached his knees,
and baggy pants with crumpled cuffs. He sat like a kid,

with one foot hooked around the other ankle. And when he hung up the phone and crossed the room, he walked like a child, taking large steps and not moving his shoulders.

"Since I've been watching the disease in this city [New York]," Sonnebend said, "it never occurred to me—never seemed possible—that this disease could be a specific syndrome, a new infectious agent," a single virus acting alone. "The patients getting sick had been exposed to an extremely complicated biological environment"—which *was* new.

"There has never been such a concentration of homosexual men," Sonnebend said, "because only recently have there been cities this large."

And only recently has homosexuality become socially acceptable enough for there to be an efflorescence of the fast-track gay life-style. It couldn't be a coincidence, Sonnebend believed, that the cities with the greatest number of AIDS cases had the most active sexual scene. The men coming down with AIDS typically had been exposed to a number of different diseases and immunosuppressors: gonorrhea, CMV, EBV, gay bowel syndrome, semen. The obvious question that struck Sonnebend was not how someone exposed to that environment could get sick but "how he could remain healthy."

Like Drew, Sonnebend believed that a new virus by itself was not enough to account for AIDS. Co-factors were necessary, perhaps a disease model that involved repeated infections and interactions among various pathogens. The model he drew for me—a chart as complex as a pre-Copernican view of the universe—began with the fact of promiscuity. Which is why many gays reject his theory.

"There are some gay men who see sexual liberation, coming out of the closet, in terms of promiscuity," Sonnebend said. Any indication that promiscuity is responsible for AIDS was a threat to their identity as gay men.

Straight scientists' hostility to Sonnebend's model came not just from what seemed to Sonnebend an irrational "emotional" commitment to the single virus/single disease theory but also from other implications of the multifactorial theory. If the multifactorial theory is true, anyone with constant assaults on his or her immune system would be liable to get AIDS, including people living in unhygienic conditions or suffering from poor nutrition—people in slums and in third-world countries.

Sonnebend believes AIDS is common among the poor around the world.

"The most common cause of pneumocystis is malnutrition," he said.

He suspects that AIDS may have been a leading cause of death among the babies of Vietnamese refugees, and that AIDS may exist in Bermuda and in the Dominican Republic. He started listing places around the world that may have had outbreaks of AIDS.

"If I could get a simple grant, a small one of only $10,000 to go around the world, I'm sure we'd find AIDS all over," he said.

But even in this country, he can't get access to the evidence he needs.

"I suggested doing autopsies on drug addicts [looking for AIDS]," he said, "but [the authorities] resisted it, because it would suggest that they'd missed it."

We may be missing evidence of AIDS among the poor and dispossessed because they are invisible. Their deaths are below the scientific and media horizon of the Western world. Who does an analysis of T-cell ratios among the dying in the streets of Calcutta? Who does a tissue analysis, looking for *pneumocystic carinii* pneumonia, of the lungs of the dead in the villages of Mali?

A paper on AIDS, co-authored by Sonnebend, Witkin, and David T. Purtilo, a doctor at the University of Nebraska Medical Center in Omaha, pointed out, "In any group, unless suspected, pneumocystis pneumonia will not be detected, as its diagnosis requires biopsy and special stains in most patients."

In other words, if you don't look for AIDS, you might not find it; and if you don't want to find it—in the third world and in slums—you simply avoid looking for it. The diagnosis becomes, to some extent, a self-fulfilling prophecy.

If AIDS is epidemic among the wretched and the forgotten of the world—if AIDS is caused by malnutrition and miserable living conditions—"to make people well," Sonnebend said, "it is not enough to set up clinics, but you must eradicate poverty, hunger, and filthy ghettos," which is harder than writing a prescription for an antibiotic. Not to eliminate the root causes of the disease in the slums and the third world while trying to cure those in the middle class who have it would be an admission that health is a luxury reserved for the rich.

4.

The American champion of the single-factor theory is Dr. Robert C. Gallo, of the National Institutes of Health, where he is chief of the National Cancer Institute's Laboratory of Tumor Cell Biology. In the late seventies he was the first to identify a virus responsible for human cancer, and a few years ago he reported that his cancer discovery, a retrovirus called HTLV-1 (the initials stand for *human T-cell leukemia virus*), might be the cause of AIDS.

At about the same time French researchers at the Pasteur Institute in Paris were announcing the preliminary results of their work with their candidate for the cause of AIDS, a retrovirus they called LAV (for *lymphadenopathy-associated virus*).

Clearly both laboratories were neck and neck in their research.

In the spring of 1984 rumors about a major breakthrough—and about increased competition between the Pasteur Institute and the National Cancer Institute—began circulating. Word leaked that the Pasteur Institute was about to make a stronger claim that LAV was the cause of AIDS.

On Friday, April 20, *The New York Times* reported that the head of the Pasteur Institute AIDS research group had said, "I'm convinced it [LAV] has a role in AIDS."

LAV showed up in 80 to 90 percent of the American AIDS patients whose blood they had screened.

The same day, undercuting the French claim, the NIH announced that on Monday, April 23, it would hold a news conference to report on a new virus Gallo had identified, HTLV-3, antibody to which showed up in forty-three of forty-nine AIDS patients—about 89 percent. In the general population HTLV-3 antibody appears in about 0.5 percent.

The Pasteur Institute and the NIH were playing a name game. Both LAV and HTLV-3 couldn't be the single cause of AIDS unless they were the same virus. Further research into the genetic codes of HTLV-3 and LAV proved they were.

The Pasteur Institute had given the virus a new name to emphasize its claim as the discoverer. Gallo, by calling the virus HTLV-3, seemed to underline how similar it was to HTLV-1, which gave him precedence: the virus was only a variant of his earlier discovery. But to make HTLV-3 an accurate name for the AIDS virus, what HTLV stood for had to change from *human T-cell leukemia virus* to *human T-lymphotropic retrovirus.*

On Saturday, April 21, the day after the Gallo-NIH news conference was announced, Dr. James O. Mason, the head of the CDC, stated that he believed the French had discovered the cause of AIDS.

"We cannot know for sure now that the LAV virus is the agent that causes AIDS," Mason said, "but the pattern it follows in the human body makes us believe it is."

The announcement preempted any news that might come from Gallo and the NIH on Monday.

By one o'clock in the afternoon on Monday, the scramble to see who would be first to get credit for discovering the cause of AIDS had become a joke among the journalists gathered in the first-floor auditorium of the Humphrey Building in Washington, D.C., who were comparing it to a story that broke that morning about conflicting claims over $422,000 found in a Hagerstown, Maryland, motel.

"At least no one in that case is trying to pretend he wants to get the dough for the sake of humankind," one reporter said.

Although the government and the scientists were trying to pretend there was no rivalry, either between the Pasteur Institute and the NIH or between the NIH and the CDC, every denial included a grab for the credit.

The press conference opening statement by Margaret M. Heckler, then secretary of Health and Human Services, was embarrassingly jingoistic. She gave a nod to "other discoveries . . . in different laboratories—even in different parts of the world"—the *even* tinged with wide-eyed wonder that laboratories "in different parts of the world" could compete with American know-how. She *even* mentioned the Pasteur Institute, but the glory was reserved for the home team.

"Today," said her speech, "we add another miracle to the long honor roll of American medicine and science."

"If LAV and HTLV-3 are the same," said a reporter, "all they're announcing is that they've confirmed the French work."

"Remember the old jokes about how the Soviets kept claiming they discovered everything—the telephone, the electric light, the airplane—first," said another reporter. "That's what this reminds me of. Me-too science. It doesn't count if it's discovered by a foreigner."

The auditorium was about the size of a theater in a church basement, which made the crush of reporters and media technicians seem greater than it was. There were so many microphones bristling in front of the podium, it looked like an architectural detail from the spaceship in *Alien*.

"Everybody—gay and straight—is tired of reading about guys who are dying," said a reporter. "But this—a cure—this is news."

HTLV-3/LAV wasn't a cure; it wasn't even a definite cause; but it would be widely reported as such. In the straight press very few news organizations would get the story right. One that did, National Public Radio's evening news program, "All Things Considered," cautioned the public not to misunderstand the implications of the announcement. And *The New York Times* ran an editorial pointing out: "The commotion [surrounding the news conference] indicates a fierce—and premature—fight for credit between scientists and bureaucratic sponsors of research. . . . What you are hearing is not yet a public benefit but a private competition—for fame, prizes, new research funds."

Most newspapers and radio and television news shows featured pictures of Gallo and photographs of the virus, which looked like a diagram of a golf green, and reported the news as Margaret Heckler's "miracle . . . of American medicine and science." As a result, all over the country gays, lulled into a false security, thought what a friend (who used to be promiscuous, having fifteen encounters in a single night, and who in the AIDS era had become virtually celibate) said when he heard about the announcement on the radio: "Back to the baths."

One reporter at the news conference asked, "How many deaths do you think this announcement will cause?"

5.

When Gallo was introduced, he approached the podium like the only kid in the school assembly to have won a National Merit Scholarship. He was fastidiously dressed. None of Sonnebend's ratty sweaters and baggy slacks for him. He wore aviator glasses, a Hollywood touch; and his hair was rumpled, but just enough to make it look as if he had recently emerged from handling a crisis. His manner seemed condescending, as though he were The Keeper of Secrets obliged to deal with a world of lesser mortals.

At the podium Gallo started by repeating a denial that there had ever been "any fights or controversy" between his group and the Pasteur Institute.

"There was some misunderstanding while I was away," he said. "If what they identified . . . a year ago is the same as what we now have produced more than fifty isolates of and in mass production and in detailed characterization—"

His enthusiasm for his own work nearly carried him away. "—If it turns out to be the same," he said, "then I certainly will say so, and I will say so with them in a collaboration."

"Damn nice of him to offer to share credit with the people who beat him by a year," someone said.

What Gallo, the Henry Ford of HTLV-3, had done, which the French had not, was to develop a way of mass producing the virus protein. He'd also proved that HTLV-3 destroys T-4 cells *in vitro*.

Throughout the news conference reporters kept asking what Gallo's announcement meant for people with AIDS— without getting a satisfactory response. Finally someone said, "Dr. Gallo, if you had a patient in private practice, one of the ... currently diagnosed AIDS victims in this country, what would you tell him this discovery means—if anything—to him?"

Gallo replied, "Could somebody else answer that?"

"No," shouted the press.

The whole conference was unseemly in its rush to capitalize on Gallo's research. Public relations was at pains to present Gallo in a sympathetic light. Although all the evidence indicated that Gallo was a private man, the press ran stories about how his obsession with cancer was triggered when he was a teenager, watching his sister die of leukemia, a fairly cynical way to trade on tragedy, making another's death a footnote in the myth of a hero.

A doctor under whom Gallo trained had told me that even when Gallo was a young, relatively inexperienced scientist, he was remarkable for his self-assurance.

"You don't get to be that driven overnight," the doctor said.

But inspired scientists don't have to be likable to be effective. For every Einstein—with laugh lines around the eyes and time to talk to anyone, great or ordinary—there are a dozen Victor Frankensteins, Faustian heroes who make a virtue of not suffering fools gladly—*fool* being defined as anyone who is not in the Great Game, the attempt to strip nature and bare her secrets, science's own version of the fast-track life.

And Gallo has demonstrated humanity and sensitivity—at odds with his image as a driven man—by consistently fighting any attempt to stigmatize AIDS as a gay disease or gays as AIDS lepers.

Still, because he was the administration expert on AIDS, he was a convenient target for people who wanted to attack Reagan—sometimes unfairly and sometimes for good reason. From the beginning the Reagan Administration seemed to be using Gallo's work as a way of thumbing its nose at its critics who had been complaining that the federal government wasn't doing enough to solve the problem.

Among the critics was Congressman Ted Weiss, a New York Democrat who the previous December had issued a statement saying, "The Department of Health and Human Services has failed to adequately fund Federal efforts to fight the Acquired Immunodeficiency Syndrome (AIDS) epidemic. Tragically, funding levels for AIDS investigations have been dictated by political considerations rather than by the professional judgments of scientists and public health officials. . . ."

The CDC budget for AIDS research in the fiscal year 1983 would rise to $6.2 million; in 1984 it would rise to $13.75 million. The total budget for government AIDS research, including not only the CDC but also the NIH and the Food and Drug Administration, would be $28.7 million for 1983 and $61.5 million for 1984. By 1986 the Reagan Administration would ask for $126 million in AIDS funds, which some, like Dr. James O. Mason, then acting assistant secretary for health in the Department of Health and Human Services, would still see as dangerously low.

Other critics claim that all the money earmarked was not actually distributed and that the figures were padded by including in them many funds that would have gone to general research even if there had never been an AIDS epidemic.

During the year and a half following the news conference heralding Gallo's breakthrough, the conflict between the Pasteur Institute and the NIH would grow. In August, 1985, the French accused the Americans of stealing their research. At issue was not just fame and the Nobel Prize— but also money. In March, 1985, an AIDS blood-test kit became available. Between March and August, 1985, eleven million kits were sold. The United States got $1.5 million in royalties; France didn't get a franc.

This was for less than a half-year. Royalties could be far greater if blood testing becomes general—as it promises to do. The United States has decided to test everyone in the armed forces, and some scientists would like everyone in the country checked. Problems with such widespread testing, of course, range from protecting the identity of those tested— so that society does not ostracize someone who does not have AIDS but who tests positive for the presence of AIDS antibody—to the accuracy of the test itself.

One early version of the American blood test turned out to be so inaccurate—with a false-positive rate of as high as 40 percent—that it was virtually useless. And a report in a fall, 1985, issue of the British medical magazine *Lancet*, comparing American and French blood-test kits, found the American kit wrong—giving false positives—in nearly a quarter of its cases. The French kit was 95 percent accurate.

The test kit patent (U.S. Patent 4,520,113) listed Gallo,

but not the French researcher, Dr. Luc Montagnier, who led the team that first discovered what the CDC, avoiding the HTLV-3/LAV conflict, had begun to call simply "the AIDS virus." The French even had a receipt for a sample of the AIDS virus, signed by a doctor at the NIH. The receipt, the French claimed, prohibited Gallo and his colleagues from using the virus for anything except research purposes.

The Americans thought the French claim was "outrageous." They pointed out that the French had been unable to reproduce the virus, had refused to share information with American researchers, and had secretly applied for a European patent.

A British magazine, *New Scientist*, reported that "Evidence is now mounting that Robert C. Gallo has misclassified the virus that causes AIDS. The result . . . is that the world has ignored the true discoverers, Luc Montagnier and colleagues. . . ." A member of the Department of Haemotological Medicine at the University of Cambridge also questioned Gallo's status as discoverer of the AIDS virus.

Rumors spread about various researchers' fraud and investments of dubious propriety—and of countercharges of provinciality and obstructionism.

The *New York Native*, one of the few journals, gay or straight, that has closely followed this story, pointed out that "a higher level of security clearance is now required [for government research on AIDS], eliminating many scientists. . . . Only those people to whom Gallo personally gives the virus may work on it, and they may not give it to anyone else. [And] only papers on which Gallo is co-author may be published from work done on 'his' virus. This means that any evidence contrary to the HTLV-3 theory would remain unpublished." In an editorial Chuck Ortleb, the *New York Native*'s publisher and editor in chief, said, "If Gallo is the kind of man who would ignore others' significant breakthroughs and then falsely claim to have made the same discovery himself . . . what else would he be willing—and able—to falsify, and for whose convenience? What small, seemingly insignificant matters about the so-called AIDS virus might he also be fudging on—or overlooking completely."

The *New York Native* called the whole scandal surrounding the French-American conflict "AIDSGATE."

More important, however, than the clawing for credit was the effect the combined Gallo-Montagnier model would have on AIDS research.

"People working with retroviruses will now get the lion's share of research funds," Sonnebend said. "What happens two, three, four years down the line if retroviruses turn out not to be the cause—or not the single cause?"

Which may be the case.

In the fall of 1985, *Lancet* reported that HTLV-3 itself may be just an opportunistic infection that attacks when the immune system is depressed.

As Sonnebend said, assuming AIDS is caused by a single virus, whether it is called HTLV-3 or LAV, is "a big gamble."

6.

Unlike most viruses, which have genes made of DNA (the substance containing the genetic code, the biological legacy passed down from one generation to the next), retroviruses have genes made of RNA, a kind of mirror image of DNA. Usually genetic information is transmitted from DNA to RNA; in retroviruses the genetic information is transmitted in the reverse direction, from RNA to DNA.

Retroviruses are very adaptable. They can get inside a

cell, like a T-cell, and use that cell's DNA to replicate themselves. The T-cell then becomes a nursery—or, to use the figure of speech favored by the press in its description of the process, a factory—for an increasing number of the retroviruses, which eventually burst from the T-cell, destroying it, and spread throughout the body, each new retrovirus able to invade a new T-cell and start reproducing itself again.

"Retroviruses have been known for a long time in a variety of animal species," said Dr. Max Essex, a Harvard professor who worked with Gallo on the HTLV-AIDS research.

For example, Essex said, retroviruses cause "a disease similar to AIDS in cats."

Horses and mice can get diseases involving immunodeficiency. Monkeys are susceptible to an AIDS-like disease (called SAIDS), which was detected for the first time at the New England Regional Primate Reseach Center in Southboro, Massachusetts, in 1980, at about the same time that Drs. Michael Gottlieb and Joel Weisman were seeing the first cases of AIDS in Los Angeles. Scientists at both the New England Regional Primate Research Center and the University of California at Davis believed SAIDS to be caused by a retrovirus. There was no evidence that the animal AIDS-type diseases were transmittable to humans until the summer of 1985, when two research teams reported that they had successfully infected chimpanzees with HTLV-3/LAV, one using LAV itself and the other using blood from an AIDS patient. This was the first indication that an AIDS-type virus could affect both humans and animals.

If evidence of the virus was hard to find in humans, it could be, as Dr. Walter Dowdle, the director of the Center for Infectious Diseases at the CDC, said, because "the virus enters the bloodstream of the patient and affects certain cells. The body's immune system gets rid of it—or it becomes integrated into the cells, into the cells' DNA, just stays there with no apparent harm done."

Like shingles (*herpes zoster*), which is only chickenpox that has hidden in the nerves for years, biding its time waiting until the person is old and under stress, when it erupts, causing pain and blisters.

"With certain people," Dowdle continued, "because of host factors or other factors, the virus is stimulated. But by then the virus is no longer around in any large number," damage has already been done to the immune system, "and the patient dies of an opportunistic infection or Kaposi's sarcoma."

As another doctor said, "People die of the secondary infections. No one's ever died of AIDS."

7.

When a virus is introduced into a virgin population— one that has built up no immunity to it—it can spread with the rapidity and intensity of AIDS. Perhaps a virus originating, let's say, in Africa, where Gallo speculates AIDS began, among the African green monkeys, was picked up by Cuban troops stationed in Angola (or somewhere else) and brought back to the Western hemisphere.

Or perhaps it spread from city to city and country to country with the advent of the fast-track gay life-style. This new life-style democratically reached across the socioeconomic spectrum to the poor—who historically might carry a disease without suffering from its symptoms because, living in less hygienic conditions than the middle class and being more exposed to pathogens, they typically tend to be less susceptible to infectious diseases. The Indian division of society into castes may have developed in part as a way of maintaining immunological barriers between classes; the untouchables may have been untouchable for reasons of health.

Perhaps there is immunological sense behind long courtships and monogamy.

But any new scourge is impartial, like the messengers of God, the *mal'ak Yahweh*, the Ed McMahons to the celestial Johnny Carson: The burning bush that spoke to Moses, the angel with whom Jabob wrestled, the divine annihilator that killed the firstborn of Egypt, or the spirit that told Mary she was going to give birth to Jesus. Like the *mal'ak*, plagues are morally neutral, biological postmen who deliver the news, good or bad, love letters or bills. They don't write the letters.

And, like the *mal'ak*, plagues can even do good by being evil; Satan tested Job with God's permission to prove Job a pious man.

How one chooses to see an epidemic reflects a vision of the world as distinct as those held by the multifactorial and single agent/single disease theorists. AIDS is polluting the world's population; it is weeding the genetic garden. It is a sign from God (the homophobe's pet theory); it is random.

It is a medical disaster. Or—just because it's a sign that immunological barriers between cultures and classes are breaking down—it is the herald, no matter how ghastly, of a unified world culture, the biological equivalent of Marshall McLuhan's global village.

8.

"Many mistakenly appear to believe that there is little difference between the two theories"—the multifactorial and the single virus theories—wrote one man with AIDS. "Such a belief could not be more dangerous. The single virus theory is very attractive to those conservative forces who would like to destroy precisely those groups affected by AIDS. The single virus theory may be used to accomplish what the New Right's political efforts have thus been unable to accomplish."

A blood test for evidence of HTLV-3 could be misused—especially if the general population starts to panic about AIDS, which it may do as a result of recent research. There is evidence that HTLV-3 may be present in saliva and that there may be healthy carriers of the virus. Six percent of a random sampling of the medical personnel at one New York City hospital—presumably a nongay, nonjunkie, non-Haitian, *nonrisk group*—had antibody to HTLV-3. All those tested seemed in good health. None were told of the test results, because the hospital didn't want to cause a panic.

Although only 8 percent of the people with AIDS in America are heterosexuals—and only 1 percent are heterosexuals who have become infected with the disease through sexual acts—there is some evidence, especially in Africa and Haiti, that AIDS is capable of spreading to the general population. As Gallo warned, it is a mistake to see AIDS as a gay disease. Diseases don't have sexual preference.

If people come to believe, rationally or not, that AIDS could bloom into a general epidemic, that no one is free of risk, how would the country protect itself? Test everyone suspect for evidence of HTLV-3—whether they are healthy carriers or sick—and place them in quarantine centers?

Or better yet: fill the quarantine centers with anyone in a high-risk group whether or not their blood shows evidence of HTLV-3? Hemophiliacs and people who need transfusions would be exempted because the blood they get could be certified AIDS-free. But the others—the gays, the junkies, the prostitutes; all of whom are on the margins of society (or perceived as such)—could be rounded up and held against their will *for the general welfare.*

Paranoia?

"The categories we defined as risk groups are sociological categories," said Dr. Celso Bianco of the New York Blood Center. "We simply expect to find a medical or biological marker and then transplant that to a social category. It would almost . . . [be doing] the same thing the Germans did in the Second World War. Eugenics. Saying everyone who is a Jew is bad because he is a Jew and because he has the genetic traits of a Jew."

Misused, the evidence of HTLV-3 could become the AIDS yellow star.

6 / Uncivil Rights

All that could conceal their distempers did it, to prevent their neighbors shunning and refusing to converse with them, and also to prevent authority shutting up their houses; which, though not yet practiced, yet was threatened, and people were extremely terrified at the thoughts of it.

—Daniel Defoe,
A Journal of the Plague Year

1.

"I T was never just about sex," said the man with AIDS. His lips were chalky, as if he'd been drinking Gelusil and had forgotten to wipe his mouth. His eyes were red rimmed. His skin had the transparency of the paper used to cover pictures in old books; it looked as if you could peel it away to reveal more clearly another, hidden face underneath. "I enjoyed the sex, but going to the baths was also political."

Gays were hit by AIDS just when it seemed that the fight for gay rights was being won.

The gay liberation movement started in June, 1969, when the police raided a Greenwich Village gay bar called the Stonewall, and the patrons, especially the fringe groups, the transvestites and the effeminate types, fought back.

At the beginning there were two major gay organizations, the Gay Liberation Front (GLF) and the Gay Activists Alliance (GAA).

The Gay Liberation Front, which had both male and female members, was a child of the sixties, leftists, against all oppression, and committed to feminism, gay sex, and gay culture. It wanted to promote gay liberation by radical transformation of the entire social structure.

The Gay Activists Alliance had more limited aims. It

didn't want to change society. It just wanted to fight for gay rights. And *gay rights* came to mean *fucking and sucking as much as you wanted.*

"We were going to show the straight world what it was missing," one gay leader said. "We were going to show them how liberating sex was. We defined ourselves by our cocks."

Morals were seen as chains to be broken; just as, in some sadomasochistic games, chains were seen as symbols of freedom, proof that one was not limited by straight, middle-class morality. The more one fucked—and the more eccentric the manner of fucking—the freer one was. Extreme sexual arousal promised transcendent states of consciousness, the annihilation of time and space that happens when you come. Orgasm plucks you out of the here-and-now—even if only for a moment; sexual abandon attempts to extend that moment. Orgies are not about sex but about time and space. Repeated orgasms—desire rising and falling like a sine wave—trigger changes in our perception of time; the tangle of bodies, the confusion of legs and arms—whose hand is that? whose foot? whose crotch?—destroys our sense of self. Orgies are totalitarian; the participants trade their individuality for a corporate identity. They become part of a machine made of flesh, which mass produces arousal, an assembly line of sex. Orgies are, to change the metaphor, the erotic equivalent of a particle accelerator, creating an enormous amount of erotic energy that is used to break down normal states of emotion, allowing the participants to examine the basic laws of sexuality.

Fast-track gays—or straights—were seeking William Blake's Palace of Wisdom by following the Road of Excess

The quest—like Dorothy's for Oz or Galahad's for the Holy Grail—is risky. The more valuable the goal, the greater the danger. As one masochist told me, appropriating the language of the gym to the language of sin, "No pain, no gain."

If fast track gays—and straights experimenting with ill-defined political-spiritual-erotic liberation—saw themselves as pioneers, like pioneers, they had to be tough.

What they wanted was sex, not love. Friction. Orgasms. No effeminate mooning after pale youths. If you had to moon, don't yearn; drop your trousers and show your ass.

To rid themselves of the stigma of effeminate love, they did the emotional—and political—equivalent of what Davy Crockett did to rid himself of an unwanted passion. He swallowed a thunderbolt. The lightning shot through him with such force it tore off his breeches. And his guts were so hot that for weeks he could eat his steak raw and let it cook on the way down.

Tough.

American homosexuals were cultivating the macho stereotype—the biker-lumberjack-Hemingway tough guy—that straight men, under the influence of feminism, were abandoning. Giving up promiscuous sex meant giving up a hard-won *positive* identity, going back to the Nellie stereotype—even, for some, mistakenly believing that the disease was a punishment for their sexual preference.

"It would be a complete rejection of everything being gay has stood for for fifteen years," said Larry Kramer, the novelist and playwright, one of the founders of Gay Men's Health Crisis, the first AIDS support group in the country.

But, Kramer said, "You cannot do what we have done all these years and not get in trouble."

When Kramer was an undergraduate at Yale twenty years ago, he said, "The worst thing you could get was crabs. I remember, when I got my first case, I thought the world had come to an end. All right, the next thing was VD, either syphilis or gonorrhea. So you could get a shot for that. Then came hepatitis. Already, you're getting into trouble. I've got hepatitis B in my bloodstream for the rest of my life. Then there were amebas. You couldn't go to a party without everybody trading ameba stories."

That epidemic ran from the mid-1970s and still continues.

"The gay doctors just kept treating us and treating us," Kramer said. "No one ever said, 'Cool it, fellas.' "

For a few AIDS took on a fatal attraction. If they hadn't come out of the closet, it forced the issue.

"When I got AIDS," a gay man said, "it was like my body was telling me I had to take a stand."

But, for most, it added fear on fear.

In 1981 Kramer met in his living room with a group of other gay men who were concerned about the new "homosexual" disease. Three of Kramer's friends had died from AIDS; the others, too, all had friends who were dying or dead. Every month the list would get longer. They decided to throw a benefit, which was held on April 9, 1982, at Paradise Garage. Two thousand people attended, and the organizers raised $50,000. No one in the group that organized the benefit—the group that would become Gay Men's Health Crisis—realized the scope of what they eventually would have to do. They figured the existing gay health organizations would step in to deal with the disease. And so would the government.

"We thought the mayor and the health department would do everything," Kramer said.

After all, New York City has more gays than anywhere else in the world, potentially a powerful voting block. In San Francisco, which also has a large gay community, Mayor Diane Feinstein, allocated $4 million for AIDS in 1983. Kramer felt New York should be at least as generous.

But when GMHC leaders tried to arrange a meeting with Mayor Ed Koch, Koch's liaison to the gay community—who was also the liaison to the Hasidic Jewish community—kept putting them off.

He said: *The gay community in New York is invisible: I can't see you. A fire goes out in a furnace of a school on the Upper West Side, and we get three thousand telephone calls in one afternoon. How many gays are calling to complain about the city's slow response to AIDS?*

For a year and a half Kramer and his colleagues in the gay community sought unsuccessfully to meet with Mayor Koch. (The mayor's office disagrees with this version of the story.) Kramer said that they telephoned; they sent messages by way of friends in the administration. Kramer also drafted a strong letter to Koch, which was signed by seventy concerned individuals and organizations, urging the mayor to meet with them to discuss AIDS.

"There was silence," Kramer said. "The mayor's office claimed it never received it. So we sent another. More silence. We said that if we didn't get a response by a certain date, we weren't sure the community could contain itself."

This was not a tactic that would be bound to meet with success.

It didn't. The deadline passed.

Kramer had heard a rumor that the mayor's office had called an aide back from a vacation in Rio and told him to shut Kramer up. According to Kramer, four members of the board of Gay Men's Health Crisis—like the aide—owed their jobs to the mayor. The tensions at Gay Men's Health Crisis were getting worse.

Kramer and his colleagues got a former associate of Dr. Martin Luther King, Jr., to train them in techniques of civil disobedience. They planned to picket a meeting on

AIDS at Lenox Hill Hospital that had been called by Kramer's doctor, Kevin Cahill, a straight man who was one of the first to recognize the seriousness of the disease. It would be a high-level, serious affair. Even Cardinal Cooke had agreed to attend the meeting. The mayor would also be there.

The day of the meeting, it poured. Kramer wanted three thousand protesters. A few hundred promised to show up. About thirty came.

The mayor's aide who had said of the homosexual community *We can't see you* was right. Politically, gays were invisible. Kramer thought they were through.

But all the television stations covered the picket. The next morning the mayor's office called Kramer's group to arrange a meeting.

There was, however, one condition: Only ten emissaries from the gay community could attend the meeting, two from Gay Men's Health Crisis, which was the group Kramer assumed he'd represent.

The Gay Men's Health Crisis board was composed of upwardly mobile gays who had not all been politically active in the past (one member of the Gay Men's Health Crisis board is even still in the closet); and it tended to distance itself from the scruffier, more radical, more outspoken elements in the movement. As its representatives to the mayor's meeting, it selected the president and the executive director.

Kramer had been frozen out.

"I couldn't believe it," Kramer said. "I'd been the driving force behind the organization. For a year and a half I'd devoted every waking hour to working for GMHC and getting a meeting with the mayor—and now I wasn't going to be one of the representatives. I said, 'I go, or I quit.' It was dumb politically of me to do it that way. They accepted my resignation. I felt like Moses—I'd led them to the Promised Land, but couldn't enter myself."

Kramer's anger at GMHC is shared by others.

"The only thing GMHC wanted people with AIDS to do was to be 'performing bears'—to go on at the end [of a fund-raising event], make them cry, and then pass the hat," said one gay leader with AIDS. "Many of us found this extremely patronizing."

Other AIDS support organizations have had short lives—like the AIDS Network, which was started by Kramer to include those who felt ostracized by Gay Men's Health Crisis. But none could compete with Gay Men's Health Crisis, which, for better or worse, remained the primary source of AIDS support in New York City.

The mayor's office set up a task force that included scientists and representatives from various concerned agencies and that met regularly with members of the gay community to discuss problems—an organization Kramer dismissed as being so bogged down in bureaucracy it is "a farce."

Red tape did tangle up plans that were heralded as triumphs of civic compassion. Even the $1.2 million Red Cross contract to provide AIDS patients with home care—at one time the largest AIDS program in New York—helped only seven patients in the first six months of operation.

Kramer continued to point out such outrages—and continued to alienate gay leaders who were working with the city. Increasingly he was seen by the GMHC board as too strident, a political liability, an embarrassment to the gay community.

He raised issues others wanted to ignore, including a tendency among some gay men to seek risks and to define themselves by their sexuality. If you define yourself principally by your sexual behavior, what happens when your sexual behavior becomes fatal? If, faced with AIDS, you become celibate, indulging in no sex acts, gay or straight, are you still homosexual? Is homosexuality just behavior, as Gore Vidal suggests; are there no homosexuals, just homosexual acts? Is homosexuality an attitude, a perception of reality, a genetic imperative, a sociological whim, or a psychological disposition?

Recent research by the dean of American sexologists, William Masters, has found that gays frequently have fantasies involving straight sex and straights frequently have fantasies involving gay sex. Is a gay who dreams of fucking a woman a latent heterosexual?

If fantasies don't define your sexual orientation and you aren't engaging in homosexual acts, what then makes you homosexual?

Kramer saw homosexuality as "a culture that," he said, "includes Proust and Tchaikovsky, John Maynard Keynes and da Vinci and Michelangelo. *I* am not going to be defined by my cock."

Kramer thought that "on some basic level a lot of people are ashamed of being gay. It takes guts to tell your parents, march in a parade, go to dinner with your lover."

Instead, too many gays haunt the precincts of anonymous sex.

"What kind of existence is it, fucking around like we do?" Kramer said. "That's why there's so little love among gay men. There's a whole segment of gay sex that gets off on the dangerous—doing it in the open and in subway johns, which I find reprehensible," he said. "I will not go to the barricades fighting for a man's right to have sex in the subway johns. But you're not supposed to say that. Whenever I make a lot of noise, I get it from the gay community."

"Read anything by Kramer closely," said a letter to the *New York Native*. "I think you'll find the subtext is always: The wages of gay sin are death."

"Just like in the Jewish community, you're supposed to keep silent," Kramer said. *"Don't say anything bad about the Jews. Don't say anything bad about gays.* Only now looking back on it can we see how dumb, blind, and dangerous that was."

In 1978, three years before AIDS was officially recognized, Kramer published a novel, *Faggots,* which by describing one weekend odyssey into gay sex, from the baths to the bars to Fire Island, confronted what was happening to the gay community. In it he showed how American homosexuals were, as he said, "Fucking themselves to death."

"I meant it spiritually," Kramer said. "It came true literally."

The reaction was—using the comparison Kramer makes of Jews and homosexuals—comparable to the reaction Philip Roth got when he published *Goodbye, Columbus.* He was vilified, virtually excommunicated. By the gay leaders.

Among the rank and file, the book was popular. Kramer received over three thousand letters from gay men thanking him for telling the truth.

"That's when I began to see," Kramer said, "the mass is not spoken for by the leadership."

AIDS had increased this gap. "Because of this epidemic, twenty-five million people"—American homosexuals—"are becoming more and more invisible," Kramer said. "An epidemic of death, instead of pulling us together, is pushing us back into the closet. I am ashamed of my fellow gay man. He's become the sissy every straight man always said he was."

2.

Like Bianco, Kramer draws a comparison between the position of Jews in Nazi Germany and that of homosexuals in America in the era of AIDS.

At about the same time that he quit Gay Men's Health Crisis, Kramer visited Munich, Germany.

"I saw Dachau," he said. "I noticed that it was started in 1933. I said, 'Where the fuck was everybody back then? You can't keep something like that secret. Why didn't somebody do something?' And I'm not talking about the Germans. I'm talking about the Jews. I came back to New York and started doing some research. It's funny: If you ask American Jews, 'Did you know about the concentration camps?' you get the same answer that you get when you ask the same question in Germany. Everyone says they didn't know what was going on."

Kramer's office is filled with books on the Holocaust and with documents on AIDS. He leaned against his desk, a momentary pause. While talking about AIDS, he'd been in constant motion, digging out copies of letters and clippings, flipping through books for references.

"A commission headed by former Supreme Court Justice Arthur Goldberg, which included former Senator Jacob Javits, Senator Abraham Ribicoff, and [psychologist] Bruno Bettelheim, issued a report which answered the questions: Did the American Jewish community know about the Nazi concentration camps and could they have done anything about them?" Kramer continued. "The answer to both questions is an emphatic *yes*."

But the Jewish community was fragmented—rich Jews and poor Jews, Sephardic and Ashkenazi, urban and rural, Northern and Southern, Republican and Democratic, members of the American Jewish Committee and of the American Jewish Congress.

"Everyone was at each other's throat," Kramer said. "The parallels with gays in America, today, are obvious. And it's appalling because we had great leaders back then—Hans Morgenthau, Felix Frankfurter, Bernard Baruch, Rabbi Stephen Wise. But they all said—like Wise did—*I know Roosevelt. I'll talk to him behind the scenes. Let's keep it quiet. We'll work from within.* And they failed. This report says over and over again, working from within doesn't work, it never works, you must not be co-opted by the system. The only way you can get any results is to fight."

Kramer quoted from the Goldberg report:

> The record showed that Allied governments were well aware of Hitler's extermination policy but for a variety of reasons were generally reticent and evasive about calling attention to the fact that his target was genocide of the Jews. They made little or no attempt until very late in the war to rescue Jews and in some cases actually obstructed such attempts by others. Their attitude on the subject was construed by the Nazi authorities as tantamount to acquiescence. Goebbels [the Nazi propaganda minister] in his diaries wrote, "At the bottom I believe both the English and Americans are happy that we are exterminating the Jewish riff-raff."

Kramer also took a tour of the United States to see how various cities were handling the AIDS crisis. He'd just written an article—"1,112 And Counting"—for the *New York Native*, which was being republished widely and was creating national controversy. It began: "If this article doesn't scare the shit out of you, we're in real trouble. . . ."

Kramer was playing Paul Revere, alerting a sleeping populace to danger. The article had profound impact in gay communities around the country, especially in cities where, because there were few or no AIDS cases, the crisis had been invisible.

When he got back to New York, Kramer started writing a play about his experiences of the last few years—*The Normal Heart,* which Joseph Papp produced at the New York Shakespeare Festival in 1985. Although ostensibly about AIDS, it is related to the disease the way Arthur Miller's play *The Crucible* is related to the McCarthy era and the way Albert Camus's novel *The Plague* is related to fascism. The play is about Jews in Nazi Germany as well as about AIDS, about prejudice and love, about the nature of power and powerlessness.

The action begins in a doctor's office in July 1981, when people were first learning about AIDS. During a physical examination Ned Weeks, a character based on Kramer, asks his doctor, Emma Brookner, "What's happening?"

"All I know is this disease is the most insidious killer I've ever seen or studied or heard about. And I'm afraid it is on the rampage," Brookner says. "And I think we're seeing only the tip of the iceberg. I'm frightened nobody important is going to give a damn, because it seems to be happening mostly to gay men. Who cares if a faggot dies. Does it occur to you to do anything about it?"

"What about the Mayor?" Weeks asks. "The Health Department?"

"You have a Commissioner of Health who got burned with the Swine Flu epidemic," Brookner says, "declaring an emergency when there wasn't one. You have a mayor who's a bachelor and I assume afraid of being perceived as too friendly to anyone gay. And who is out to protect a billion-dollar-a-year tourist industry. He's not about to tell the world there's an epidemic menacing his city. And don't ask me about the President."

"Do you realize you are talking about millions and millions of men who have singled out promiscuity to be their principal political agenda, the one they'd die before abandoning?" Weeks says. "How do you deal with that?"

"Tell them," Brookner says, "they may die."

3.

I stayed up until three in the morning reading an early version of the play.

"No more making love?" a character—Ned's lover—who has just been diagnosed as having AIDS asks Dr. Brookner.

"Right," Brookner says. "Unh, I guess if you use condoms."

"Hey," Ned's lover says, "I get to wear my rubbers again."

"Sorry," Brookner says. "That's the best I can do."

"Want to hear a golden oldie?" Ned's lover says. "Using a rubber is like washing your feet with your socks on. Did you hear the one about the condom and the carrot? The carrot says to the condom: 'Boy, what a shitty life I've had. I'm so mistreated. I get ripped out of the earth, I get yanked from my bunch, they pull out my green hair by the roots, I get stripped of my skin by a sharp knife, I get cut into quarters, and then I get drowned in a dip.' The condom replies: 'You think you got it bad? Some guy gets inside me, pokes me in a dark hole, does a hundred push-ups, throws up, and faints.' "

Joking in the face of death is a way of both challenging

and deferring to a power greater than your own—like King David dancing before God. A valiant gesture.

Later on another character chides Weeks for being so outspoken: "I . . . just don't think you should tell people how to live?"

"Drop that! Just drop that!" Weeks says. "The cases are still doubling every six months." Of course we have to tell people how to live! Or else there won't be any people left!"

In the version of the play I read the word *AIDS* is not mentioned once.

When I read it, I'd been researching AIDS for nearly a year, and I'd reached the point at which the stories I heard, no matter how pitiful, struck me merely as material. In fact, the more heartrending the tale, the better copy it would make.

Kramer's play managed to strip away my cynicism—partly by scaring me. I began contorting myself in order to look at the soles of my feet for purple blotches, telltale signs of Kaposi's—the AIDS scarlet letter, which, like Hawthorne's, starts as a sign of sin and ends as a badge of martyrdom.

Maybe I'd picked up AIDS in a laboratory or crisis center. Although at the beginning of my research I'd been fastidious, using a handkerchief over doorknobs in laboratories—even in gay organizations—by the end of my research I'd gotten immune to the fear of the disease.

Now, after reading Kramer's play, I realized how strung out I'd gotten in the research. There was a period when I'd be home just long enough to catch a night's sleep before flying off for another series of interviews. I was so exhausted that once I left Los Angeles for Houston, where I was supposed to talk with people at the KS/AIDS Foundation; conked out during the flight; woke just long enough to get off the plane and into a cab and tell the driver to take me to the downtown Regency; dozed again; and woke just as the taxi was pulling up to a hotel that didn't look like it was downtown.

"Is this the Regency in Houston?" I asked.

"Mack," the driver said, "this is the Regency in Denver."

Listening to tapes of AIDS interviews, I realized I'd had a bad cough for weeks. Maybe I was getting pneumocystis pneumonia?

My family doctor was unavailable, so I went for a checkup with the physician who was covering. He treated me with an odd manner, which betrayed contempt and disgust. Obviously he had been getting closet gays who were afraid they had AIDS but were ashamed to go to their own doctors, and he thought I was one.

"I'm just writing on AIDS," I said.

He looked up at me over the top of his glasses and said, "Yeah."

But Kramer's play didn't just scare me, it placed AIDS back into a human context. When I saw a production of *The Normal Heart,* the audience was filled with older men and women, defeated-looking suburban couples who did not look like the kind of people who usually went to off-Broadway plays—presumably parents of gay men, possibly gay men with AIDS. The stage was between two facing rows of seats. Halfway through the first act I glanced up from the actors and saw couple after couple wiping tears from their eyes. They were no longer audience; they were witnesses. They'd become part of the play's action.

When I started my research, I taped to the wall over my desk a quote from one of the first AIDS patients I'd interviewed—something that had begun to seem like a platitude, something that hit me anew with its original force when I sat down to make some notes on my reaction to the play:

"Imagine what it would be like to find out that making love could be fatal."

4.

Fear and compassion. Of the two reactions to AIDS, I suspect fear would dominate if AIDS began to spread widely into the straight community. Among liberals—who might be expected to support a movement like gay liberation but who have never rallied around that cause with anything like the fervor seen in other comparable causes— AIDS offered an excuse for what seemed to be political apathy but what was in fact fear of sexual contagion: If you support gay liberation, someone might mistake you for a gay.

When I went to an AIDS benefit at New York's Symphony Space in the spring of 1984, I couldn't get any friends to attend—people who were usually ready to come to the aid of any good cause.

"Aren't you afraid to be seen there?" one asked me.

The crowd was filled with gay stereotypes: clones and thugs in black leather jackets. Outside the theater two bums were hanging around.

"What's that?" the first asked.

"They all got GAIDS," the second said.

"What's that?" the first asked.

"Like cancer," the second said. "They all gonna die."

"Let's go over there," said the first, pointing across the street, apparently overwhelmed by the prospect of all that death.

There were posters for the previous year's benefits—the performance of Ringling Brothers' Barnum and Bailey Circus at Madison Square Garden in April, 1983, and the rodeo in October—AIDS T-shirts, stamp-out-AIDS buttons.

"Collectors items," shouted a guy hawking them, relegating AIDS and AIDS items to a past in which AIDS is no more than a memory. Instant nostalgia.

"The country shuffled off the Depression by watching Ethel Merman on Broadway," said the emcee onstage, introducing the evening's entertainment of songs from the thirties. More nostalgia.

The past seemed safer than the present. In the thirties homosexuality was hidden enough for it to surface as a café-society style. You didn't have to anguish over whether or not to come out of the closet because no one was coming out of the closet. And AIDS did not exist.

In *Illness As Metaphor,* Susan Sontag analyzed how a disease can be perceived as expressing a historical period. Tuberculosis becoming a symbol for the early Industrial Age; cancer, for our own time. AIDS draws some of its fascination from the same process: It seems to sum up a sensibility. It is the ultimate vulnerability for men who have made themselves emotionally vulnerable. At its worse, it, like many diseases, offers its sufferers secondary benefits: the they'll-be-sorry-once-I'm-gone temptation to demand attention from others. It lets people who feel like victims act out their internal script in a horrible way. Like Jenny Wren, who in Dickens's *Our Mutual Friend* goes up to the roof to pretend to be dead. Or like pseudo-Camilles, who have spent years swooning in various imaginary romantic deathbed scenes, which have now become the real—and tragic—thing. This kind of exploitation of a disease is not unique to people with AIDS, gay or straight.

At its best—if a fatal illness can be said to have a best—it gives people a spiritual whack on the side of the head; makes them understand what may be the hardest thing for anyone alive to grasp: We all are mortal, so we'd better do what we want to, do what we must. Many gays with AIDS are able, because of the seriousness of their condition, to put aside festering family resentments and reach out to their parents; many parents are able to put aside their anger and hostility and let their sons know how much they love them.

This may have helped give the night a feeling of possibility and hope.

Or maybe it was just the giddiness of people partying on the brink, as they did in the thirties, as they're doing today. The sense of imminent apocalypse, whether it is due to AIDS or war, the Depression or the Bomb, makes life not only dangerous but also heroic, as though everyone in the audience were on a doomed ship, sailing off into the night with its band playing and its lights blazing.

"I'm a gay man with AIDS," Michael Callen was saying onstage, "and singing is what I used to do before I got sick. But I'm better now, and I'm back singing."

The audience went wild with applause.

There was a whiff of disinfectant in the air, something I'd smelled in the same theater when I'd taken my daughter there to see the Paper Bag Players; but now it had sinister associations: hospital corridors and sickbeds.

Callen explained that the song he was going to perform was about survival.

"Oh, what dumb luck I just had," he sang.

5.

"The question was who needs panda?"

The quote was tacked to a bulletin board in the old offices of Gay Men's Health Crisis, a cramped brownstone, decorated with a stuffed koala and teddy bears hugging each other, pictures of pandas, panda quotes—"Better butt on small pandas."—a poster used in AIDS literature of two naked men, one white and one black, embracing, with the tag, "You can have fun and be safe too," and a newspaper clip with the headline: *Homo Nest Raided.*

Gay Men's Health Crisis pioneered AIDS support services, like its outreach programs, which included a hot line (that in the spring of 1985 was answering about three thousand calls a week), crisis intervention counseling, group therapy, a recreation program (offering everything from museum trips to writing classes), and financial counseling. The last was a crucial service, since having AIDS can be expensive. Medical costs for a person with AIDS runs an average of $140,000; the cost of treating the first fifty AIDS patients at one New York hospital was about $3 million; and the national cost for AIDS care may reach $30 billion in the next five years.

Many people with AIDS, who don't fall under the strict CDC definition, may not be able to get government help like Medicaid in paying their bills. And private insurance companies are considering excluding AIDS from coverage if the applicant does not take an AIDS blood test.

But the most successful service Gay Men's Health Crisis established was their "buddies" program, in which volunteers—Gay Men's Health Crisis has close to one thousand volunteers working in various capacities—help people with AIDS, shopping for them, cleaning their apartments, being generally available to do what needs to be done.

Gay Men's Health Crisis also offers legal advice.

"There are particular legal problems that gay people face in this epidemic that nongay people wouldn't face," said the Gay Men's Health Crisis president, who prefers that his name not be used, an extraordinary scruple in an organization that seems to believe no one should be ashamed of being gay.

"If you were sick in a hospital and were nongay," he said, "your wife would have no problem visiting you. But a gay man's lover is not considered family, and he might have trouble getting in to see the patient. A lot of nongay lawyers are not even aware of the potential problems."

Gay Men's Health Crisis also tries to make sure the patient's will is proof against challenges, since many parents will try to prevent their son's lover from inheriting anything.

"A dying gay man will suddenly have his parents arrive out of nowhere because they are next of kin," said Judy Kreston, a New York therapist who has done a lot of AIDS counseling. "And the lover is shunted aside."

To hide the truth at funeral services, some parents will try to pass off a woman as their son's girlfriend.

Parents see death as a way of reclaiming their wayward children—as though being gay were like joining a cult and death were the ultimate deprogrammer.

"Some parents who really can't stand the idea that their son is gay see the disease as a bad news/good news situation," said another therapist. "You know: 'The bad news is your son is gay. The good news is that he's dying.' "

6.

After New York the city hardest hit by AIDS has been San Francisco, whose gay community—from 20 percent to 40 percent of the population, depending on whose estimates you trust—is among the most visible in the country. The epidemic took root there in 1982, when physicians began seeing gay men with Kaposi's sarcoma.

"[The disease] was starting to get a lot of press play, stuff like *Gay Plague Strikes Homosexual Community,* that sort of thing," said Ed Powers, one of the leaders of the AIDS Foundation.

For a short time the police wore anti-AIDS masks. People, both gay and straight, warned each other not to eat in restaurants. Who knew how AIDS was transmitted; who knew which cooks and waiters were gay? Gay men who were known to have AIDS were thrown out of bars. Something had to be done to reassure and educate the public.

Marcus Conant, a dermatologist who was the first doctor to report a case of Kaposi's and who in 1985 was the chairman of the California State Task Force on AIDS; Cleve Jones, a gay activist; and some other concerned people put on a public forum to inform people about the strange disease. This led to the creation of the Kaposi's Sarcoma Research and Education Foundation, which became the AIDS/KS Foundation and later the San Francisco AIDS Foundation.

At the time the only other AIDS group in the country was New York's Gay Men's Health Crisis.

"With a little bit of money that was raised," Powers said, "we opened up an office on Castro Street," the heart of the gay ghetto. "There was one desk, one telephone, no chairs, a few pieces of paper and a couple of pencils."

As the months passed, there was a flood of volunteers. The group published a brochure listing AIDS symptoms, how to find a doctor who knew about the disease, and basic risk reduction information.

Powers sat in the AIDS Foundation's new offices on Tenth Street, in a room that was nearly as bare as the original office, except this simplicity was a reflection of elegance, not poverty. On the wall of the office were safe-sex posters. One—"An ounce of prevention"—had eleven suggestions for escaping AIDS, like "Know your partner, his state of health, his lifestyle, and how many different sexual partners he has. If you enjoy being with a partner, see him again." Another said: "Sex is an important part of our lives. We owe it to ourselves and to our partners to keep it as healthy (low risk) as we can." That redefinition of *health* from its traditional meaning ("absence of disease") to "low risk," made being well merely a matter of a gamble. Which, in fact, it probably is.

"Originally the idea behind the organization was to set up chapters throughout the country, to provide information and raise money that would be funneled to a central board that would [in turn] fund research," Powers said. "One of the things that quickly became apparent was that the national idea wasn't going to work because local communities wanted to form their own organizations. Another thing that quickly became apparent was that the kind of research necessary [to find the cause of and cure for AIDS] can only be funded by the federal government."

Some of the founders of the organization held on to the dream of a national organization; others, like Powers, wanted to focus their attention closer to home. The group split. And the faction Powers belonged to became the AIDS Foundation.

At around that time Powers saw a man who was suffering from a disease rare even among people with AIDS: cryptosporidiosis. Its principal symptom is severe diarrhea, which can lead to malnutrition. It is caused by a protozoan and is found usually in calves.

"He had applied for social security," Powers said, "and had been told by the disability determination officers that the disease he had was only found in animals, therefore he couldn't have it, therefore he couldn't be disabled, therefore he couldn't have SSI [social security insurance]."

Powers went to Congressman Philip Burton. Burton went to Washington, fought the Social Security department, and got Social Security to acknowledge that AIDS—in all its protean manifestations—is a debilitating and disabling disease.

That was a watershed case. The AIDS Foundation began working more and more on advocacy—particularly since another organization in San Francisco, the Shanti Project, was offering patient services like New York's Gay Men's Health Crisis's "buddy" program.

7.

In the outer office of the Shanti Project, a volunteer was talking on the hot line to someone about a sad case, a man with pneumocystis who was stranded and abandoned: "If he's home and can't walk, he'll need attendant care. This should have been taken care of before he was released. The doctors are rampantly incredible about sending people home before they belong at home. Or without proper care. Now, it's very hard at a distance for you—or me, for that matter—to know what is necessary, much less ideal."

His tone was calm, but there were tears in his eyes.

The Shanti Project was founded in 1974 to provide emotional support and peer counseling for people with life-threatening illnesses and their loved ones. Originally the project dealt mostly with cancer patients, some people with heart conditions, and similar diseases. In 1984 it was located in a community center, the Pride Center, which looks like a Masonic temple, the clubhouse of a secret brotherhood. In the inner office Jim Geary, the director of the project, sat dressed in a white Indian-style smock, bright blue slacks, and a multicolor necklace. His feet were bare. On his wall was a sign that said: *AIDS: Anger to Action.*

When Geary joined the Shanti Project six years ago, he was one of the few gay men on the staff. The project's first AIDS-related activity was a support group that Geary started in his living room in November of 1981, when there were only about thirty diagnosed cases of AIDS in the city. The following year the Shanti Project lost its funding; the board of directors resigned and turned the project over to the volunteers; and the project focused increasingly on AIDS. In December of 1982 the city of San Francisco decided to support the project. In 1984 the city gave $412,000. In 1985 Shanti planned to ask for an additional $150,000. And they expected to get at least another $150,000 in donations.

By February of 1984 the project's board of directors decided to limit its services to people with AIDS and their families and friends. Shanti had grown so large it had, in 1985, over 300 volunteers, who each worked for about eight hours a week. And as of the spring of 1985, it had served over 750 people with AIDS and over 3,000 of their family members and lovers.

For counselors, Geary said, "We look for people who are sensitive, who can listen nonjudgmentally, who don't have their own agendas."

Along with the expected patient services, by early 1985 the project had three group homes, each housing four to five people with AIDS who can't afford to pay rent or who have been evicted from their homes—"frequently," Geary said, "by their roommates," who are afraid of contracting the disease. More group homes were planned.

"We work a lot with the issue of sexuality and the changes that our clients need to make," Geary said.

That is the hot topic. It divides itself into two key issues: compulsive sexuality and safe sex.

Compulsive sexuality. The erotic equivalent of eating salted peanuts. Once you've put sex at the center of your identity—whether you say "I am a gay man" or "I am a straight stud"—you need a constant series of sexual adventures, each one upping the ante of the others, in order to nourish your sense of self. What happens when that need slams up against your instinct for survival?

After years of indulging in sex for sex's sake, it's hard to break the habit. The brain's pleasure centers are used to being stimulated; like rabid hyenas, they howl and gnash their synaptical teeth when they are not fed. But pleasure can become a taskmaster; it can be as ruthless as guilt. If the purpose of sex is pleasure, you can become obliged to have the most exquisite pleasure possible or feel you have wasted the encounter.

If you add to that the newly revived Elizabethan notion that sex can cause death, that every orgasm brings you closer to the grave, you have the makings of a first-rate compulsion as exciting as risking your life savings on one roll of the dice. In fact, more exciting. The greater the stakes, the greater the risk. And the greater the risk, the greater your focus of attention. And in sex the closer attention you pay to the moment, the greater your arousal.

At the other extreme, gay men, seeking shelter from the storm of sex and disease, have taken refuge in drugs that block their sex drive. They have tried vitamins and herbs, psychoneuroimmunology counseling, and stress-reduction seminars. Or they have joined AA-type groups: When the urge hits, they call a friend who talks them down.

The goal of treatment is not to "cure" the person, but rather to have him keep up his fighting spirit in the face of chronic "illness." [Wrote a New York physician, R. William Wedin, in the *New York Native*]: Why does such a pessimistic philosophy have such a broad appeal? . . . There is something very *American* in the whole idea of fighting shoulder to shoulder, and side by side, against the forces of evil—be they the Indians, the Communists, the demon rum, or gay "promiscuity." To be sure . . . one may have to use all sorts of scientific-sounding jargon . . . and scientific-looking "logs" of one's sexual experiences . . . to make the old-time religion sell. But even in the high-drag of science, it is all still there—the moralism, the righteous aggression, the comradeship in arms—*the works*. . . . Never mind that one's career and/or social life is falling apart from spending every free moment watching porn on the VCR. So long as one is staying out of the baths and backrooms, one is presumably doing O.K.

Some have joined clubs that give their members sexual driver's licenses: guarantees that they all are AIDS-free. But since the disease has such a long incubation period, that remains a hit-or-miss solution. A few have retreated into willful celibacy, which has developed a whole philosophy (not just among gay men but also among straight men and women who are afraid of herpes and other venereal diseases). Many gay men go to neither the extreme of courting danger out of compulsive sexuality nor of avoiding danger through chastity. They compromise: They still go to the baths but they only jerk others off, masturbate themselves, or watch.

"Men and women have not been used to thinking about periodic abstinence—especially coming out of the late sixties and the early seventies, when a freer, more active sexuality was considered to be a right," said one psychologist. "As a result, many people, especially from their mid-twenties to late thirties, have profound problems with the idea.

They want to have intercourse when they want to have intercourse."

When they can't fuck, they throw the erotic version of a tantrum.

But many cultures have periods of enforced abstinence, the awed and awful sacrifice of pleasure to the mysterious forces of generation. In the quest of rationalism—our impossible grail—our culture has shed one sexual taboo after another in a kind of intellectual striptease. We make few sacrifices to the elemental powers of creation, and who knows what unpurged poisons pool in our psyches and seep into our souls because we avoid the discipline of periodic abstinence. Freer sexuality does not necessarily mean more exquisite sex; it may, in fact, make us jaded. Just compare the keen thrill of teenage petting, *touching bare skin for the first time,* to the blunted pleasures of, for the heterosexual, going to a sex club like Plato's Retreat on a regular basis or, for the homosexual, going every week to a bathhouse. Maybe the unappeased gods doom us to being equally unappeased, unsatisfied.

We have to reeducate ourselves in the advantages of taboos and learn what is known by cultures that have periods of enforced abstinence. One man said that on the days he chooses not to make love, "I feel tremendously energetic. I feel more powerful. It's just a matter of learning the trick of not feeling like you're getting cheated."

The division in the gay community between the orgiasts and the celibates has focused on the question of whether or not to close backroom sex bars and bathhouses. The conflict went public in an article, titled "Whitewash," published in *California Magazine.* This, said Powers, "basically quoted a lot of people accusing everyone else gay in the city of being murderers or criminally negligent, because the leaders of the gay community had not gotten up and told gay men to stop having sex."

The bathhouse issue inflamed tempers. Gradually, the community was ripped apart, split between followers of two San Francisco gay organizations—the Harvey Milk Gay Democratic Club (which made the charge) and the Alice Club. Any hope of united action to deal with the crisis was quickly vanishing.

Candlelight marches are a traditional way of demonstrating gay solidarity. One man with AIDS, Gary Walsh, suggested to Powers that they might bring the community back together by staging a march in memory of all the men who had died of AIDS and to demand that Washington do something about the epidemic. Powers called Larry Kramer and suggested that New York stage a march on the same night. Kramer called the National Gay Task Force, an organization that theoretically speaks for America's gay population, with the idea. And on Monday, May 2, 1983, candlelight marches with the theme "Fighting for Our Lives" were held in twelve cities.

"I thought we'd have maybe five hundred people [in San Francisco]," Powers said. "The five hundred we expected showed up, and they brought about nine thousand five hundred friends with them."

New York had about the same number marching. Altogether the national turnout was about twenty-five thousand.

"As we were coming down Market Street, there was a little hill," Powers said. "I looked back. All you could see for about a mile and a half, almost all the way back to Castro Street, was a line of people with candles."

But that wasn't enough to keep the community from splitting.

8.

Every day the conflict between those who wanted to keep the bathhouses open and those who wanted them closed sharpened. During the summer of 1984 there was even a case in which a gay man in a New York City bathhouse was recognized as a person with AIDS, ostracized by the other men there, and finally run off the premises. Because the debate involved social, sexual, and political issues, it became a focus of concern, a litmus test: What you believed about the bathhouses identified you.

The issue was unnecessarily and unfortunately narrowing to a fight between health and civil rights.

7 / The Double Bind

Because of their forced isolation from society, lepers' legal identities became muddled. . . .

—Robert S. Gottfried,
The Black Death: Natural and Human Disaster in Medieval Europe

1.

"OUT of the tubs and into the shrubs," men in towels shouted as Dr. Mervyn Silverman, then San Francisco's public health director, announced on April 9, 1984, the decision to ban sexual activity in the city's gay bathhouses.

"The existence of bathhouses, whose sole purpose is to facilitate multiple, anonymous contacts, runs counter to controlling the spread of AIDS," Silverman said.

The ban would be enforced the same way the health department policed its hotel and restaurant regulations—through the use of unannounced visits. The ban, however, was not put into effect until six months later, when fourteen bathhouses were closed.

Silverman moved against the bathhouses after fifty prominent gays signed a petition demanding action. In a poll of gay men in the city, 52 percent wanted to ban sex in the baths—or close them down. If Silverman had resisted, the very people whose civil rights he might be threatening would attack him.

That was only one of the manifestations of the paradox he was faced with. If he didn't respond to AIDS as a gay issue, he would be accused of not recognizing gay needs and thus of being hostile to the gay community. If he did respond to AIDS as a gay issue, he would be accused of being prejudiced.

He first came up against this bind when he started an extensive AIDS education program—by the summer of 1985 the city had given out over a half-million pamphlets—aimed at educating the providers of health care, the general public, and the gay community. Gays were leery of the plan.

According to some gays in San Francisco, at least a few of the fifty gay leaders who had signed the petition to Silverman felt, at least in retrospect, that they had been tricked into doing so. Gays opposed to the closing of the bathhouses claimed that another poll, run by the San Francisco Department of Public Health and the University of California (San Francisco) showed that 74 percent of gay males were not in favor of Silverman's action—an action some gays saw as an attempt by a mayor who was hostile to gays to keep the bathhouse issue from being voted on.

Those gays believed closing the baths was insensitive, medically unsound, and based on a condescending, homophobic, and perhaps even unconstitutional attempt to modify behavior.

"There is so much fear in the gay community about the rise of homophobia, [about] things that would cause the successes in gay liberation to be lost," Silverman said.

A fairly innocuous poster that told gays not to share bodily fluids, use condoms, avoid recreational drugs, and to "enjoy more time with fewer partners" was booed at a national gay health conference in Denver. You weren't supposed to call public attention to the gay community—especially not with posters that connected gay sex to AIDS. How would the straight public react?

By August of 1984 the groups that wanted to keep open
the baths got support from San Francisco's Human Rights
Commission, which voted unanimously to oppose "any action by the City . . . to close bathhouses or prohibit or regu-
late private consensual sexual activity in any bathhouse or
sex establishment, absent a showing that it is a necessary
and essential public health measure supported by clear and
convincing medical and epidemiological evidence."

A few months later, when fourteen gay sex clubs and
bathhouses that had been closed defiantly reopened, Silverman attacked them for putting greed above concern, accusing them of being "establishments which . . . profit from
the spread of AIDS." A logical leap: The sex clubs and
baths don't profit from AIDS; they profit from anonymous
and promiscuous sex, which, in turn, might spread AIDS. A
subtle, but significant, nuance.

"From a legal perspective, such drastic government intervention to control sexual conduct would set a precedent
in endangering the fundamental right to privacy of all gay
people irrespective of where such conduct occurs," Meriel
Burtle, one of the attorneys representing the baths, was reported as saying. "How do we stop the . . . prohibition of
consensual sexual activity in one location [from becoming a
prohibition of] . . . such activity in all locations?"

2.

"The anxiety level in the gay community peaked," Silverman said, just as the anxiety level of the straight community started to climb. Straights were panicked by the
prospect of getting AIDS from casual contact. The more
they were told not to worry, the more worried the straights

got, because, as Silverman said, people naturally distrust the government, which, after all, says, "Don't worry about Three Mile Island. Don't worry about Love Canal."

How could the straights trust any statement about what's safe and what's not safe? How could the gays trust the government not to act on the fears of the majority?

In July of 1983 the city opened the world's only AIDS unit in a local hospital, which isolated the people with AIDS, protecting them from infections they might contract in a general ward and giving them the kind of concentrated medical attention they might not otherwise enjoy. A lot of people, both gay and straight, were convinced that this was an attempt to quarantine the people with AIDS—the precursor of AIDS concentration camps.

How could anyone suspect such authoritarian behavior in San Francisco, a city noted for its tolerance?

Tolerance, even in San Francisco, may not be as deep as we'd like to believe. Prejudice festers right under the civic skin.

When I left the city, my flight back to New York was delayed, and the airline lost my reservation.

"What a way to run a business!" I said in disgust.

The woman at the counter, annoyed at my annoyance, said, "Another pushy Jew from New York, huh!"

3.

For governments, passing laws that seek to control private behavior is the legislative equivalent of designing a house. Since we've started, why not add one more bedroom. And an extra bath. How about a deck. With a hot tub. And a solarium. A gazebo out back. A tennis court! In for a penny, in for a pound. Once you start, it's hard to stop. Lord Acton was half right: Power does corrupt; but absolute power doesn't corrupt absolutely. It justifies.

It's a small step from closing baths to regulating sexual activity, no matter where it occurs. This was demonstrated when the bathhouse controversy heated up in New York City in the fall of 1985.

The debate raged not just between factions of the gay community but also within the straight community. And the bathhouse issue was fueled by behavior not in sex clubs but in schools.

The stage was set in the middle of June, 1985, when Dr. Arye Rubinstein of the Albert Einstein College of Medicine in the Bronx testified before the New York City Council Committee on Health. He estimated that in New York as many as three hundred children had AIDS or AIDS Related Complex, and over a period of a year, as many as seven hundred babies with AIDS could be born in the city.

Nationwide, by the beginning of September, 1985, there had been 165 reported cases of AIDS in children twelve years old or under; 113 had died. There were an additional 61 cases of AIDS in adolescents between thirteen and nineteen years old.

Most children got the disease *in utero;* some were infected by the mother's blood during delivery; a few may have contracted the disease through breast-feeding. About 20 percent got AIDS through transfusions. A small number of the adolescents were infected through sexual contact and shared needles.

"The numbers are increasing now and the rate is much steeper than has been seen in other populations before," Rubinstein said. "People do not realize the magnitude of the problem."

Not long afterward the wire services picked up news of a thirteen-year-old Kokomo, Indiana, boy with AIDS. He was a hemophiliac who had been infected through a transfusion of tainted blood. Afraid he would spread the disease to other students, local school officials refused to let him enroll in the seventh grade at Western Middle School. They arranged a special telephone link with his classroom.

By the fall of 1985 AIDS in the classroom had become an issue, especially in New York, New Jersey, Connecticut (New Haven authorities barred two children, one with AIDS and the other with AIDS Related Complex, from schools), California (where children with AIDS would not be allowed in classrooms), Indiana, Massachusetts (in Swansea an eighth-grade boy, a hemophiliac who got AIDS from a transfusion of contaminated blood, would be the first American child with the disease to be allowed to go to school), Florida (three sisters, triplets, with AIDS attended first grade in an isolated classroom, where they were instructed by a volunteer teacher), and the District of Columbia.

Even communities that had no children with AIDS were troubled.

But in schools the danger was to children with AIDS who might die from the normal childhood diseases, which their classmates would shake off in a matter of days. Given everything known about AIDS, there was virtually no threat to healthy, uninfected children.

But the public was titillated by the connection between kids and a fatal disease that was spread principally through homosexual sex acts. It hinted at a connection between innocence and vice.

Politics is a form of magic: The audience fools itself and gives the credit to the magician. Since parents were scared about AIDS in schools, politicians had to respond—especially politicians in New York, the American city with the largest number of AIDS cases. By the summer of 1985 New York City had over 4,300 cases, about a third of all the cases reported in the country. At least 400,000 New Yorkers had been exposed to the virus. And in New York more men between twenty-five and forty-four died of AIDS than from any other disease.

Because of numbers, New York City was willy-nilly a test case. What happened there could hint at what might happen next year or the year after in the rest of the country.

And the city's AIDS program was in trouble.

"I don't think the city has any real intention of providing educational services [on AIDS]," said Pat Mar, who in July, 1985, quit her job as coordinator of AIDS education. City officials, she said, "definitely want to keep AIDS quiet."

No wonder parents were uninformed and confused about the risk kids with AIDS posed to their classmates.

At a parochial school—Holy Name—on the Upper West Side, parents threatened to withdraw their children from classes when the New York Archdiocese decided to house AIDS patients in an adjoining building. The archdiocese backed down.

In the public schools the battle was fiercer.

By the fall of 1985 seventy-seven New York City children had AIDS. Half had died. Seven, all eight years old or younger, were of school age; four of them might attend school.

Even though two local doctors who specialized in treating children with AIDS—Larry Bernstein and Brian Novick, both from Albert Einstein College of Medicine—and the CDC assured city officials that it was safe for the infected kids to be in the classroom, two of the city's thirty-two school boards rebelled.

The two districts—district 27, the largest in the city, and district 29—were both in Queens, working-class neighborhoods of single-family homes, median incomes above the New York City average. Some of the areas are unreachable by subway. According to one of the district officers, this kept them isolated, "a lot like . . . the 1950s," protected from the social changes that occurred during the past quarter-century in Manhattan: drugs, the sexual revolution, gay liberation. In many ways these districts were more representative of the rest of America than were Manhattan or San Francisco.

The two districts said they would defy any order from the schools chancellor, Nathan Quinones, that allowed kids with AIDS into the schools.

Quinones tried to finesse the issue by saying the kids with AIDS were too sick to attend classes. And Mayor Edward Koch said the decision whether or not to allow the kids with AIDS to go to school would be made on a case-by-case basis.

"I don't believe it's healthy for the AIDS kids or for the other children," Koch said. He predicted, "I don't believe you're going to have any kids with AIDS ending up in the classroom."

Three children were kept out of school. Two were in hospitals, where they would be tutored. One would be taught at home.

A fourth child, a seven-year-old second-grade girl whose symptoms were in remission, would be allowed to attend classes.

"This child is no danger—no danger—to other children," Koch said. "You can panic if you want to, but I hope you won't."

People panicked.

On the first day of school eleven thousand to twelve thousand students boycotted classes. Kids picketed with signs like *No children with AIDS in any of our grades.* On the second day of school nine thousand students stayed home.

Parents warned their kids not to kiss other kids, not to share food or clothing. Rumors spread that at least ten people who had taught in the city's schools had AIDS. The schools chancellor finally announced that eight people, including teachers, administrators, and one food service employee—a cook at a Brooklyn school—had AIDS. Three of them, including the cook, had died the previous year.

Parents worried about whether the cook had cut himself, bleeding into the food their children ate. The schools chancellor explained AIDS was not transmitted through food.

Stranger scenarios were suggested. What if a kid with AIDS spit into another student's face, into his eyes or mouth? What if a kid with AIDS bled into another student's open wound? What if a kid with AIDS bit another student?

Such worries were unreasonable. Despite some researchers' suggestions that AIDS could be transmitted through prolonged, intimate kissing, the virus did not appear in high enough concentrations in saliva to be a threat. There was not a single case of AIDS being transmitted through biting, sneezing, or close sibling contact. Nor did the virus appear in high enough concentrations in tears, so a kid with AIDS was unlikely to transmit the disease by weeping on another kid, one fear expressed by parents. And the virus did not seem to be present in sweat, urine, or feces.

There was no evidence you could get AIDS from a swimming pool, toilet seat, silverware or plates, showers or locker rooms. Eventually the American Academy of Pediatrics would announce, "The risk of acquiring AIDS among children is low. There has been no instance whatever of child-to-child transmission."

Still, Queens School Board 27 brought the issue to court.

In mid-September Dr. Ronald Rosenblatt, who had treated over one hundred people with AIDS, said he thought letting a child with AIDS go to school was "medically unsound."

Dr. Lionel Resnick, an AIDS researcher at Mt. Sinai Medical Center in Miami, Florida, said, "I'd take the conservative approach and not expose the child to other children" because, among other reasons, the immune systems of young children are not fully developed.

A few days later the governor of New York, Mario Cuomo, said that although the children with AIDS were "entitled to a little compassion," he would be "scared to death" to send his fifteen-year-old son to school if one of his schoolmates had AIDS.

"We have to recognize that people are right to be afraid," he said.

He said he wanted the state health commissioner, Dr. David Axelrod, to "tell the people of the state all he knows" about AIDS.

Mayor Koch established a new panel to decide whether or not students with AIDS should be allowed in the classroom; the head of pediatric AIDS studies for New York City's health department announced that as many as two thousand students in the public school system could be carrying the AIDS virus; and the whole issue was clouded by confusion when it turned out that while the seven-year-old girl at the center of the controversy had been infected by the AIDS virus, she did not have AIDS.

The whole drama was a reflection of how the country was responding to AIDS: a crisis over misinformation.

4.

At the same time that the AIDS school controversy raged, experts were predicting that by 1990 virtually every child on earth would be vaccinated for measles, tetanus, whooping cough, polio, tuberculosis, and diphtheria. And on a slow day for AIDS news, the *New York Post* ran a scare headline: *Protect Toddlers From Killer Disease: Mom.* The disease was Haemophilus B, a rare illness that kills one out of every twenty affected infants and that every year strikes about a hundred times more kids than have reportedly contracted AIDS since 1979.

Childhood disease was becoming a hot topic.

It was a development of the country's dread of children, which had been exploited ever since *The Exorcist.* Now kids were possessed not by the Devil but by Death. This is a self-serving myth that comforts an aging baby-boom generation, which—having overvalued youth in the sixties (*Don't trust anyone over thirty*)—now must undervalue youth in order to feel that it's okay to grow old.

As for Governor Cuomo's request that New York State Health Commissioner David Axelrod "tell the people of the state all he knows" about AIDS. . . .

On October 25, 1985, Axelrod said there was no doubt that AIDS was spread by anal and oral sex.

He asked the state Public Health Council to vote on a sixty-day emergency regulation, which would allow local health officials to close gay bathhouses and other places, like peep shows, porno theaters, and adult bookstores, where people engaged in high-risk sex.

"We think that some state action is welcome, but we still

have serious reservations regarding essential civil liberties," said Ron Najman, a spokesman for the National Gay Task Force. "We cannot condone the state prohibiting private behavior between consenting adults."

"It's a regulation of shocking overbreadth," Tom Stoddard, the legislative director of the New York Civil Liberties Union, was reported as saying. "This regulation purports to outlaw any form of nontraditional sex between any people outside the home. It goes way beyond the issue of AIDS."

How could such a regulation be implemented?

How do you decide that a sex act considered likely to spread AIDS is taking place? What constitutes probable cause? When health officials suspect that such acts are occurring, what do they do?

Use ladders? reporters asked the mayor. Or periscopes? Koch replied, "You're getting into the nitty-gritty, here."

New York City stressed the importance of voluntary cooperation—gays in bathhouses avoiding unsafe sex and, presumably, reminding others. *Excuse me; stop buggering that guy. You may be infecting him.* But privately most people recognized that this was an unrealistic hope.

Even though a spokesman for Axelrod said, "We don't want . . . to go around with sex police," the ban would have to be enforced by undercover city health inspectors.

"I would think that unannounced visits with some frequency would be . . . likely," said Jean Cropper, New York City's deputy health commissioner for environmental affairs.

It all reminded one gay man of the efforts of United States Navy undercover agents a half-century ago, who engaged in gay sex acts to entrap homosexuals in the service.

Eventually Axelrod would even say investigators could "go into" hotel rooms to stop unsafe sex.

"It's an attempt to reestablish the old sodomy laws," said a gay activist. And it affected not just gays but straights, too. "If some straight married couple are in a hotel and the wife wants to give her husband a blowjob, the Sex Cops could barge in and stop them!"

Even New York City's health commissioner, David Sencer, admitted that closing the bathhouses would "contribute little if anything to the control of AIDS. . . ."

"If everyone hadn't gotten so hysterical over that one kid, who didn't even have AIDS," one gay activist said, "they never could have gotten the public to put up with that [bathhouse] ruling."

5.

The increasing hysteria over AIDS in the schools offered a counterpoint to the attempt to close the bathhouses, an effort that started at about the same time the parents in Queens were preparing to boycott the schools.

On September 23 some Christian and Jewish religious leaders, including Pastor Jesse Lee, of the Family Defense Coalition and the Neighborhood Church, and Rabbi Yehuda Levin, who was running for mayor of New York, demonstrated outside the New St. Mark's Baths, demanding that it and eleven other gay bathhouses in the city be shut down until researchers found a cure for AIDS.

"We will continue to march into the dead of winter if necessary to get the mayor's attention . . . ," Pastor Lee was reported as saying.

In response, a spokesman for the health department said, "We're not in business to close businesses."

The city would not interfere with the bathhouses.

About a week later Diane McGrath, who, like Rabbi

Levin, was running for mayor of New York, raised the ante, called for the closing of not just the bathhouses but also gay bars, gay porno theaters, and gay peep shows. Preempting any complaints that such action might be unconstitutional, McGrath said, "The AIDS virus has no civil rights."

People who harbored the virus were, apparently, no more than vehicles for a pathogen that had been raised to the status of citizen only to be stripped of a citizen's prerogatives.

The mayor and the health department still resisted closing bathhouses, or any other action limiting the rights of people infected with AIDS.

"If you want to quarantine every person capable of transmitting AIDS, you have to quarantine a quarter-million people," Mayor Koch said. "That is simply not possible."

In the first week of October the mayor had apparently changed his mind. He asked the city health commissioner to reexamine whether or not the bathhouses should be closed. And the governor, emphasizing that the decision to close bathhouses "has nothing to do with morality or promiscuous behavior," justified his position by pointing out that in the 1950s swimming pools were closed to stop the spread of polio—a poor analogy.

According to an article in the December, 1985, issue of *Discover*, the AIDS virus is so vulnerable that "If a sample suspended in a fluid-filled test-tube is left to stand at room temperature for 24 hours, it has only a ten percent chance of surviving." And, since the virus can be deactivated by heat, it might pose little threat in a Whirlpool bath or hot tub.

The state AIDS Advisory Council voted 6 to 1 against closing the bathhouses. And evidence was marshaled to prove that closing the bathhouses would have little effect, that San Francisco's attempt to prohibit sexual acts that might transmit AIDS had had only limited success, and that oral sex was not as significant a risk as anal sex in the transmission of AIDS.

"But they had to include oral sex," said a gay man who continued to go to bathhouses. "Otherwise they couldn't close the peep shows. There's not a lot of anal sex going on at peep shows. But the whole AIDS scare gives them a free shot. They've been trying to close the peeps for years . . . so they can gentrify Times Square. That's what the ruling is really about. Not safe sex. Real estate."

State and city officials disagreed. Cuomo repeatedly emphasized that he wanted to ban what he considered unsafe sex, not close bathhouses, which he admitted would be legally suspect and difficult to do.

"We're not seeking to close establishments," Axelrod said. "We're seeking to end dangerous sex."

The state would only close down clubs that did not enforce the ban on unsafe sex.

"My perception is that the governor is caught in a political bind," said Michael Callen, who was a member of the State AIDS Advisory Council. "He has to seem to be doing something. [And] nobody knows quite what to do."

Like Silverman in San Francisco, Cuomo was trapped. If he did nothing, he'd be attacked. If he did something, he'd be attacked.

"Who do you win with doing it this way?" he asked.

The confusion over what the government could do and wanted to do was increased because the legal and humane issues masked moral issues that everyone—publicly—agreed had no place in any discussion of AIDS. An odd—although understandable—notion.

It has become heresy to suggest that moral questions should be publicly confronted. But why shouldn't a society confront questions of morality?

The danger comes not from debate but from the belief that moral questions are legislatable. In fact, the courts, simply by addressing a moral issue, undermine morality.

Before there were laws prohibiting cruelty to animals, people were restrained from, say, beating horses by their own conscience—or, if conscience failed, by practicality. Horses were valuable; if you injured one, you were damaging your own property. Certainly some people did beat horses; but they were as irrational as someone clubbing a car that wouldn't start. It's unlikely any law would have much effect against such passion.

Even if the law did have an effect—especially if it had an effect—it removed from the individual the burden of behaving morally. The question became not *what is right?* but *what can I get away with?* As morality changed from a spiritual to a legal issue, it lost its private hold over people. Courts replaced conscience.

The fight over the bathhouses confused the moral question (*what sex acts should someone with AIDS allow himself to perform?*) with the legal question (*what is the government's responsibility in promoting public health?*).

This is why some people, gay and straight, who were appalled at promiscuous, anonymous, and brutal sex could be equally appalled at the state's attempt to curb promiscuous, anonymous, and brutal sex.

Public debate over private morality is not a bad idea.

Public enforcement of private morality is not a good idea.

6.

"The governor's trying to close the bathhouses without actually coming out and saying so," Jack Stoddard, the manager of the New St. Mark's Baths, said to a reporter.

In November, 1985, New York City closed a gay bar, the Mine Shaft, which it claimed had violated the state guidelines on safe sex.

It was a safe test case. The place smelled sour. It was crowded with men dressed like cowboys, bikers, construction workers; some wore only jockstraps, others wore nothing. *S/M demonstrations* . . . read a sign. *The Mineshaft's school for lower education.* There were gym horses, and a cross for mock crucifixions. Inspectors saw men giving and getting blowjobs, sodomizing and being sodomized. Just as some inspectors were about to enter a backroom, they reportedly heard what sounded like a whip and screams. They decided to investigate no further.

The Mine Shaft was "a notorious . . . place," according to Richard Dunne, the executive director of Gay Men's Health Crisis.

"The governor and the mayor have taken us down a slippery slope that may lead to recriminalization of private sexual conduct in general," said Thomas B. Stoddard, legislative director of the New York Civil Liberties Union.

In fact, before the end of the month the city would also close a heterosexual sex club, Plato's Retreat (for prostitution, not unsafe sex acts), and a federal official, possibly with the New York experiment in mind, would call for the closing of all gay bathhouses.

Koch insisted he was shutting the bar for the patrons'

184 / THE PLAGUE YEARS

own good, to impress on them how "suicidal" and "ridiculous" their behavior was.

"What we are saying," Koch said, "is that you can't sell death in this city and get away with it."

Trying to forestall public outrage at what might seem government's attempt to dictate morality, the city kept up a drumbeat, attacking the bathhouses for dodging taxes as not-for-profit institutions, for having mob ties, and for encouraging not merely high-risk sex but acts that the majority of the public would find repulsive—whips and chains, pain and humiliation.

But the public didn't seem repulsed. It seemed fascinated. Even amused. What exactly was *mummification,* which the Mine Shaft advertised. What was electro-torture? How did the Mine Shaft patrons use clothespins?

People avidly read descriptions of gay bathhouses and bars. Radio call-in programs, like the Les Kinsolving show, dwelt on details. People were mesmerized by the chance to—safely, by proxy—violate a taboo.

Breaking a taboo may be perverse. But it's also sexy.

The public was suddenly back in a metaphorical '53 Chevy, discovering for the first time a new, forbidden world of eroticism. Closing the baths and sex clubs was an opportunity to give the public a chance to vicariously open baths and sex clubs in their imaginations.

Even better. Since the public was merely witnessing, not participating in, unusual sexual activities, they could add to their excitement the satisfaction of feeling superior.

But the worse descriptions couldn't compete with a news item that ran at the same time about a man who broke into a farm in Westhampton, Long Island, and sexually molested a duck.

7.

"Bathhouses aren't what straight people think they are," said a gay man who likes them but, because of AIDS, has stopped going.

At their worst, he said, they can be foul, furtive meeting places, not much better than a doorway in a back alley— especially if they're run by straights, who look on with contempt. At their best, he claimed, they're more like spas, a model of what the ancient Roman baths must have been like.

The New Saint Mark's Baths in New York is recognized as one of the cleanest and safest bathhouses in the country, and so it offers a look at the phenomenon at its best.

From the outside it seems like an ordinary apartment building, neither forbidding nor prepossessing. Inside, you walk up a few steps to a vestibule, where there are windows like a cashier's in an old-fashioned bank or a ticket seller's in a movie theater. At one window you can rent a locker; at the other, a room. Even if it's crowded, like late Saturday night or Sunday afternoon, you can almost always get a locker.

If you want the guaranteed privacy of a room, you can wait in a coffee shop off the vestibule until one becomes available.

"In the old days you could wait hours for a room," said another former regular who has stopped going since the AIDS scare.

At the height of the AIDS panic, when attendance was halved, you often didn't have to wait at all. In the spring of 1985 attendance was back almost to its pre-AIDS level; people had to wait again.

"You sit, drinking coffee," said a gay man, "talking or looking embarrassed."

The first floor is dominated by a long room with lockers on either side, like a gym.

"If you get a locker," he said, "this is where you take off your clothes and put on a towel."

The key to the locker is attached to an elastic band, which you can put around your wrist or ankle.

At the far end is a lounge with leather banquettes, where you can smoke a cigarette and talk to others. To the left, behind the front office, is another lounge with mats on the floor and on raised platforms, where there used to be orgies. Since the AIDS epidemic the room is not kept as dim as in the past.

"It's not as mysterious," complained one man.

"They used to give you paper cups, the kind cole slaw comes in, filled with lubricant," another man complained. "Now they give you information and condoms."

In the basement are more lockers, a steam room, sauna, redwood benches, showers, and a pool.

On the second and third floor are rooms—cubicles just large enough for a mattress on a platform. There is a light on a dimmer. Clean sheets, an ashtray, hooks to hang your clothes.

"The baths have an etiquette," said a regular. "You can put on a towel and walk around outside or stay in the room and leave the door ajar—all the way or a little—and see who comes past. You communicate what you want through your body language. If you want to pick and choose, you might put a pillow behind your back and lean against the wall. If you're interested in the guy who stops outside and looks in, you might smile. If not, you look away. If he doesn't get the hint and starts to talk, you can hold up your hand—like stop—and he'll go away. If he's persistent, you say, 'No,' or 'I'm resting,' or 'I'm too tired.' " At a bathhouse that has a sleazier reputation than the St. Mark's "you get these old men who are desperate. Even if you say no, they still come in and grab you."

"If you're interested, you try not to show it," said another gay man who in the late spring of 1985 was still visiting the baths. "Usually you wouldn't say, 'Come in.' The guys who cruise past the rooms are shopping for merchandise. You're the merchandise."

A television set would not say to a customer, *Come on; try me.*

"An unwritten rule says you don't fuck people you know at the baths," said another man. "I guess, because if you haven't done it by then, you wouldn't. Lying down on your stomach without towels means you want to be fucked, and it doesn't much matter who does it. Because of AIDS, there's less of that now. Now, there's different behavior. Not as much fucking, sucking, and kissing. There used to be a lot of kissing. Now there's more touching and caressing. More masturbation"—individual and mutual—"and more just looking. People are hornier and doing less. It's like the old days."

A lot of gay men have given up going to the baths and spend a lot of time in homosexual and heterosexual health clubs, just to look at naked bodies in the steam rooms and showers.

"But," one man said, "in the baths, there are still some people lying on their stomachs."

"When AIDS first hit, I thought about the ethics of running a bathhouse," said Bruce Mailman, owner of the New Saint Mark's Baths. "Should I close down; should I stay open? I decided it's not the baths that are the problem."

Dr. Roger Enlow agreed. Enlow is a scientist who in the spring of 1983 gave up a career as a physician and came out of the closet to become head of the New York City Health Department's Office of Gay and Lesbian Health Concerns—and who, a year and a half later, at the end of the summer, frustrated by bureaucratic resistance, quit.

Throughout his tenure he slowly was being torn between two opposing forces—those members of the gay community who wanted to close the bathhouses and those who did not want to close the bathhouses because that would be an infringement on gays' civil rights.

Enlow leaned toward the position that closing the bathhouses would violate gays' civil rights.

"The closure of the bathhouses is not the point," he said. The point, he thought, was "how to modify behavior."

But—according to Michael Callen, who has AIDS, who founded People With AIDS/New York, and who has been on a crusade to close the bathhouses—you can't modify behavior if you leave open the institutions that encourage the very acts you want to discourage. His stand on bathhouses has made him unpopular with what he calls "the white, male, essentially conservative . . . hierarchy" of those in control of the AIDS service organizations like Gay Men's Health Crisis.

Geraldine Ferraro was, as she said, "so impressed and moved" by Callen's story that in May, 1983, she read a statement he had made into the *Congressional Record.*

He was discussing a support group he belonged to, made up of people with AIDS.

Whenever I am asked . . . what we talk about in our groups, I am struck by the intractable gulf that exists between the sick and the well. . . .

We talk about how we're going to buy food and pay rent when our savings run out.

We talk about how we are going to earn enough money to live when some of us are too sick to work.

We talk about how it feels to get fired from our jobs because of unjustified fears of raging and lethal contagion—fears based on ignorance and unfounded speculation. . . .

We talk about the pain we feel when our lovers leave us out of fear of AIDS.

We talk about the friends who have stopped calling.

We talk about what it feels like when our families refuse to visit us in the hospital because they are afraid of catching that quote "gay cancer" unquote.

We talk of what it feels like to be kept away from our nieces and nephews and the children of our friends because our own brothers and sisters and friends are afraid we'll infect their children. . . .

What we talk about is survival.

Callen is a thin man who speaks with a quiet urgency, the efficient passion of a man who has a lot to do and no energy to waste. Eighty percent of those diagnosed as having AIDS at the same time as Callen was first told he had the disease—in December, 1981—have died.

"I have thought a great deal about the issue of censorship within the gay community," he said. "I've had to, being so often the object of censorious efforts. I am torn. The party line would have it that we shouldn't wash our dirty laundry in public—that the straight press loves nothing more than to show our movement in disarray, more occupied with internal squabbles and turf battles than in getting on with the life and death business at hand. On the other hand, from speaking to gay people in other cities, I have come to realize that the majority of gay people get their information about AIDS from the *straight* media. . . . So I have decided to take my chances with the straight press in the hope that by telling my story as honestly and truthfully as possible I can reach a larger group of people and maybe make some small impact on how people think about this disease."

He believes it is imperative that people understand the role of promiscuity in the transmission of AIDS.

"It was my use of that word which . . . blocked my effectiveness as a spokesman from the beginning," Callen said. "As I have come to learn, asking a clone to take a step back and question the dogma of promiscuity is akin to walking into a fundamentalist Baptist convention and suggesting that they seriously consider the possibility that God may not in fact exist. But I am stubborn. I *hated* the gay male double standard. So . . . I pulled out all my gay books and looked up the word *promiscuity*. What I found was that if one wanted to say positive things about promiscuity, the meaning of the word was never questioned; but if one wanted to be at all critical of promiscuity—of the absurd, reductive notion put forth that promiscuity is what knits the gay community together—one was immediately attacked. . . ."

Because of gay politics, Callen was slandered—a rumor was spread that he was a Moonie. He had to resign from the AIDS Medical Foundation, and he was removed as one of the press contacts for a New York City–sponsored brochure advocating safe sex.

"People spend so much time fighting among themselves that they have little energy left to fight the real enemies," Callen said. "Who *is* the real enemy? What about the enemy within? I consider a gay Republican to be as real an enemy as any heterosexual of similar conservative political persuasion. As one gay man from South Carolina was quoted in Boston's *Gay Community News* (I'm paraphrasing), it seems to me that *gay Republican* is a contradiction in terms. I could more easily imagine rimming Jesse Helms than voting for him."

8.

If progressives—who are ready to rally to nearly every other liberal cause—have avoided coming to terms with AIDS, it's not surprising that the rest of society has not been sympathetic.

When AIDS was first detected in 1981, there wasn't much media attention; during the summer of 1983, when the fear arose that AIDS was going to spread rapidly into the straight community, there was an explosion in coverage. After the winter of 1983–1984, when, once again, it seemed the heterosexual population was safe, coverage diminished. Apparently as long as AIDS remained a threat principally to gays, the press was content to treat it as a minor story.

"If previously healthy straights were getting a fatal disease for which there was no cure and the number of cases was doubling every seven or eight months or so, the story would be in the papers every day," said a reporter. "You know, like the Iran hostages: *Day four hundred and seventy-two. So many sick, so many dead.*"

There have been some exceptions. Although the gay community faults *The New York Times* for its coverage of AIDS, many gays first heard about the disease from the *Times* in 1981; and, ever since, the *Times* coverage of the medical, political, and human stories has been regular and sensitive. In the first four months of 1984, at a time when many newspapers were cutting down on AIDS pieces, the

Times ran two dozen articles on AIDS and mentioned the disease in fourteen other articles—an average of over two stories a week, which has been typical. In the fall of 1985 the *Times* was running a story—sometimes two stories—nearly every day.

Thorough series have appeared in the *Philadelphia Inquirer, Newsday,* and the *New Haven Register.* The *Washington Post, The Wall Street Journal,* and *USA Today* have also given AIDS wide and responsible coverage. The *New Republic,* the *New York Review of Books,* and *TV Guide* have all treated AIDS in depth. *New York* has had a number of well-written, well-researched pieces on AIDS, and one moving personal account by a man who was dying of the disease. *Newsweek* and *Time* have run thoughtful pieces on the effect of AIDS on gay life-styles and on the AIDS school controversy. The *Village Voice* has run excellent articles on the politics of AIDS. And, although *California*'s famous "Whitewash" article fanned both gay and straight fears, it was an early and honest attempt to come to grips with the effect of AIDS on society. *Discover* has had a clear, well-organized piece on AIDS. Good pieces have also appeared, although sporadically, in some local newspapers like the *Sarasota* (Florida) *Herald-Trubune.* And surprisingly, *The National Enquirer,* despite some awful coverage of Rock Hudson's illness and death, has had at least one nonsensational, informative AIDS piece.

AIDS coverage has been slighted in places that should have covered the story in depth, like *Science News,* which tends to report only on the breakthroughs, and the *Los Angeles Times,* which skimps for a city with the third largest population of AIDS patients. And until recently the epidemic has been badly handled by magazines like *US* and *People,* which tended to focus in a ghoulish way on descriptions of people suffering from the disease; however, both made decent efforts to cover the effect of AIDS on Hollywood. The *New York Post* predictably exploited the disease for its shock value *(L.I. Grandma Dead of AIDS)*.

On television, the coverage on ABC's "World News Tonight" has been careful to allay panic. "The CBS Evening News" has been generally good, although at first somewhat hesitant to deal head-on with the disease. According to *TV Guide*'s News Study Group, CBS forthrightly announced that the majority of AIDS victims were male homosexuals, but it stated nearly a year later that sexual transmission was second to transmission through blood. NBC's coverage was both sensational and misleading. In describing AIDS, Tom Brokaw used loaded words like *terrifying* and *out of thin air,* and Jessica Savitch referred to AIDS as the "killer disease." NBC also reported that Dr. Anthony Fauci of the National Institutes of Health said children could pick up AIDS through routine close contact, a fact that does not seem to be borne out by research and that could easily terrify relatives and friends into unnecessarily and cruelly closing their homes to people with AIDS.

The worst coverage on television, many in both the gay and the medical communities agree, was Geraldo Rivera's "20/20" report on May 26, 1983, in which he said that AIDS had contaminated the nation's blood supply and "the safest thing to do is store up your own blood." The broadcast may have been responsible for a dangerous dropoff in blood donations.

The gay press with the exception of the *New York Native*—which deserves a Pulitzer Prize for its comprehensive coverage—hasn't been much better than the straight press. Compared to the *New York Native, The Advocate,* a national gay journal, has tended to downplay AIDS. Although some local gay newspapers (like those in Los Angeles and Denver) have been informative, most have been very cautious.

"What can you expect," said a gay activist. "In most cases gay newspapers are surviving on ads for bathhouses— where people are most likely to pick up AIDS. Too much coverage tends to cut down on bathhouse attendance, which makes the newspaper's advertisers unhappy."

9.

In the late summer of 1985, when it was announced that Rock Hudson had AIDS and when parents began worrying about AIDS in schools, the press disgraced itself in an orgy of necrophilia that was paranoid, ill informed, and obscene.

Hudson had looked wasted when he'd taped a cable television show, "Doris Day's Best Friends." Public denials— which usually precede public admissions—began appearing in late July. On the twenty-fourth, newspapers were claiming that Hudson had cancer of the liver.

According to Hudson's spokesman, Dale Olsen, one of Hudson's doctors "said there was no indication of AIDS"—a claim that in about a week was replaced by a report that Hudson not only had AIDS but would die in two months.

The obsession with whether or not Hudson had given AIDS to his television co-star in a televised kiss melted the barrier between soap opera and life. Reality began to seem like merely one more episode of "Dynasty," an episode that involved hundreds of thousands, maybe millions of people.

A few journalists treated the story responsibly, using it as a chance to inform the public—like Liz Smith, who pointed out how difficult the disease is to get and suggested that the press "stop all these 'scare' headlines and 'made-up' stories. We need massive infusions of money for research and education about AIDS," she wrote. "The government needs to get into the act to stop what is an authentic and frightening epidemic. But we don't need all this silly and inaccurate sensationalism."

But most of the press surrounded Hudson's suffering with grisly hype. *Rock on the Ropes. Rock's Gift to Liz. Doris Day Mourns Her Friend: I'll See Rock in Heaven. Fear & AIDS in Hollywood: It is a town near hysteria. More H'Wood Stars Hit with AIDS. Double Lives, and Damaged Careers. The Dynasty Kiss— Rock Hudson's Last Plea: Linda, Forgive Me!*

Like the primitive cultures that make some unfortunate man king for a day and then sacrifice him to fertility gods, Americans create heroes only to destroy them. In between we force them into Central Casting procrustean beds. The Drunk Poet, The Philandering Leading Man, The Misunderstood-and-More-Talented-Than-Anyone-Imagines Sexpot, The Macho Novelist, The Tortured Comic. Our national commedia dell'arte troupe.

Celebrity is a private club; and, as with many private clubs, it has a limited membership—a certain number of spots available. Someone has to die before a pledge is enrolled.

Which is one reason the death of a celebrity excites us. Suddenly the field is open; who will fill the old hero's shoes? Who will become the new Hemingway? The new Monroe? The new Joe Louis? The new Elvis?

The king is dead. Long live the king.

Rock Hudson was a matinee idol. A romantic leading man. That was his slot, no matter how comfortable or uncomfortable privately he may have been filling it.

The discovery that he had AIDS violated the rules of the

game. Suddenly he wasn't what we thought he was. He wasn't a great womanizer. He liked men.

At first the press and the public were stumped. Emotions were blocked. The press didn't know how to play the news. The public vacillated between outrage at Hudson's betrayal of his image and compassion.

Jokes popped up—and disturbing reminders. For a while it seemed like Hudson was about to switch roles in his last days—hero for tragic clown. Early in September, not long after news of his illness hit the press, I turned on the television. *Pillow Talk,* one of his most famous movies, was half over, and Tony Randall was asking Hudson, "What have you got against marriage anyway?"

I'd heard rumors that Hudson was gay, that he had in fact married a male lover, but I don't think I would have reacted to, even noticed, this line if Hudson's homosexuality had not been highlighted by the knowledge that he had AIDS. All the attention to his disease in a gruesome way made the line comic. That is, it made the line tragic and therefore inappropriate to the situation, juxtaposition of contraries being one of the forms of comedy. The line was comic *because* it was tragic, because the film had lost the magic barrier that separated the story on the tube from Hudson's story in life.

But myths cannot die. And the people who temporarily embody the myths are helpless to change their role, like men grown too big or too small for a suit of armor they cannot remove.

Hudson was a hero. So what if he was gay and had AIDS. He played his farewell scene heroically.

Whether or not he wanted to, he had to.

Hudson was doubly victimized—by the disease and by the public.

10.

Los Angeles was the city third hardest hit by AIDS. Despite—or perhaps because of—the homosexuals in the movie industry, it does not have a gay community that is as active or visible as the ones in New York and San Francisco, and so it has escaped both the internecine wars and paranoia that are splitting New York's and San Francisco's gay communities.

"The gay and lesbian community here want quarantine, want separate wards in hospitals," said Dr. Martin Finn, the director of the health department.

They want it because it dramatizes political recognition that the gay community is being decimated by AIDS. But the city has been resisting the demand, mostly for practical reasons. An AIDS patient with Kaposi's will be put in a cancer ward. Someone with pneumocystis will be put with other people who have pneumonia.

Probably because gays are less visible as a distinct group in Los Angeles, the AIDS Project/Los Angeles sees itself more as an AIDS center than a gay center. And in 1984 the head of social work there was a straight woman, Colleen Johnson.

Johnson has the face of an Irish saint and the stamina of a heavyweight prize fighter, and she understands the problems fear of AIDS can create, like the unwillingness of ambulances to transport people with AIDS.

"We get an incredible number of calls for transportation," she said, "because people's lovers and friends hold jobs; and if they stopped going to their jobs to take the person here and there to the thousands of doctors' appointments [someone with AIDS has], then they'd lose their jobs, and the only income coming in is cut off."

Often someone with AIDS has to wait two or three hours for an ambulance company to round up a volunteer crew. And just as often an ambulance will arrive, the crew will discover that the patient they've been called to transport has AIDS, and, Colleen said, "they'll sit out in their van and talk to their boss for fifteen minutes before they get up the guts to go in and do it."

Or they'll refuse to take the patient and will drive away.

Despite Colleen's problems with ambulance drivers, doctors, dentists, nurses, employees, and even therapists who refuse to have anything to do with people with AIDS, Colleen believes the most devastating prejudice is not institutional so much as personal. She cites case after case of AIDS patients shunned by families, friends, and business associates.

"One guy invited a friend with AIDS over for Christmas dinner," she said, "and the others who had been invited said if he came they wouldn't, so the guy with AIDS was asked not to come."

After a while the people with AIDS begin isolating themselves—like the man with AIDS who was waiting outside Colleen's office, bundled up in an overcoat in the middle of a California summer day like a character from a Gogol story. He shrank back when I entered the room. His face was cadaverous, pale as porcelain. When he yawned, I could see the roof of his mouth which was the maroon of uncooked kidneys. He had raccoon eyes, a bluish tinge as though he'd put on eye shadow and eyeliner, as though Death were making him up for some terminal night on the town.

"He used to be a body builder," said one of the workers

at the project. "The healthiest person I knew. His biceps were huge."

His coat was draped around his shrunken figure almost as loosely as it would have been around a hanger.

He was convinced he had done this to himself. It was the cost of his sins.

AIDS patients must keep in mind what Dr. Robert Krasnow, a Los Angeles therapist, said: "There are no guilty people with AIDS; there are only sick ones."

The burnout among Project workers is great. Volunteers who can't take the tragedy anymore bolt. Even one of the Project secretaries quit. When a pet cat died, one of the staff members broke down and sobbed. She was unable to stop and didn't know why. She'd loved the cat, but the reaction seemed all out of proportion. Finally she realized that these were the tears she had not allowed herself to shed for all the people with AIDS who had died.

"We try to allow people the denial they need," Colleen said. "When people give up hope, they die faster."

So if someone claims he is going to be the one to beat the disease, the workers at the Project don't tell him he is being unrealistic.

"I know they say everyone who gets it is going to die," said the lover of one AIDS patient, who had come to the Project for help, "but my friend is going to be the exception."

"We know that's probably not true," Colleen later said, "but why not let him believe it?"

While I was there, Colleen excused herself: She remembered she had to call someone with AIDS who had been getting better, someone who had become a symbol for her—and for other people at the Project—that maybe AIDS wasn't always fatal after all.

She dialed the number, listened for a moment, and said, "Oh, my God. His number's been disconnected."

"I saw him in the hospital just last week," said Dan Morin, the coordinator of Volunteer Services.

"This isn't a good sign," Colleen said.

"Don't get anxious," Morin said.

"Don't get anxious," Colleen repeated, overwhelmed by the denial she allowed others. "It's probably nothing."

Colleen told me about a man with AIDS who had given the disease to his wife. She was pregnant, and her baby was born with AIDS. The only one in the family who was healthy was their five-year-old daughter, who asked her mother, "Are you going to die?"

"Yes," the mother said.

"Is daddy going to die?"

"Yes."

"Is the new baby going to die?"

"Yes."

"Can I come with you?" the girl asked.

11.

"I keep coming back to the question: *Why me?*" said a gay man I'll call Ron.

Two weeks before I met him, he'd come down with a slight fever, which didn't go away. His lover, aware of the symptoms of AIDS, urged him to go to a doctor. The doctor told him he had AIDS—*pneumocystic carinii* pneumonia.

"He also told me I probably would die in a matter of months, maybe weeks," Ron said. "He'd treated many people with AIDS and was sick of saying encouraging things that he knew weren't true."

Ron's voice rose and fell like a radio station that is being broadcast from a distant place and keeps fading. He sat in the hospital bed in hospital pajama bottoms and a top he'd brought from home. It had a pattern of footballs and logos of football teams. A forked tube went into his nostrils.

Before entering the room the nurse asked me to put on a surgical mask.

"Is it safe?" I asked her.

"No," she said. Then, seeing my reaction, she explained, "I mean, it's not safe for him. It's safe for you. You're the one bringing in all the outside germs."

"I went through all the typical stages," Ron said. "Denial, anger, all that. Now, I'm just stunned. Like I've been mugged. I mean, I was never promiscuous. No more than any heterosexual. In five years I've had maybe two, three lovers. They weren't that promiscuous either. So why me?"

The speech tired him. He lay back, his mouth open, his eyes fixed on some point above my head. There was a long silence.

Finally he said, "Aren't you going to ask the question?"

"What question?" I said.

"What's it feel like to die?" He looked at me. "You don't really understand, do you, that probably by the time your [book] comes out, I won't be here to read it."

12.

In America in the fall of 1985 there were over 13,000 officially documented AIDS cases. About half of the afflicted—over 6,750—had died. If cases continue to increase at the same rate as in the past few years, there could be 26,000 cases in 1986, which means that by the beginning of 1987, 13,000 people could be dead from AIDS.

Sixty to 120,000 other Americans may have AIDS Related Complex (ARC), a milder form of the disease that seems to develop into AIDS in 10 to 20 percent of the cases. And the number of Americans who, while not yet diagnosed as having AIDS or AIDS Related Complex, may be infected with the virus is—according to current government estimates—500,000 to over a million. Former New York City Health Commissioner Dr. David Sencer estimated that just in New York City there are about 400,000 gays and drug abusers infected with AIDS. All figures—both the estimates for New York City and for the whole country—may be twice or even ten times greater.

At least 25 percent of that infected one million will probably get AIDS Related Complex, and 10 to 20 percent of those with ARC will probably get full-blown AIDS. That could mean over 20,000 cases. And if the statistics remain the same, one percent of these cases will be presumably transmitted through heterosexual sex acts: That means 200 new cases of AIDS among a so-called nonrisk group.

If the rate of increase remains what it has been.

But the rate of increase in AIDS cases seems to be slowing.

When I first started researching AIDS two and a half years ago, the number of cases was doubling every six months. As I write now, at the end of 1985, it takes about a year for the number of cases to double.

Not only has AIDS *not* begun spreading through sexual contact among the heterosexual population at a faster rate than it did in the past—it has maintained a one percent share of the cases—it also seems to be slowing slightly among gays. Facts that few in the media or scientific community have publicized—possibly because it seems in almost everyone's interest to feed fear.

The media can capitalize on fear to panic people into

buying more newspapers and tuning in to more news shows. Scientists can profit from fear because it puts pressure on the government to award larger research grants. The government can use fear as an excuse to increase social control, and politicians either in or out of office can take advantage of fear to get headlines and votes. Gays can exploit fear to force the straight community to concern itself with a disease that otherwise might be dismissed—in fact, for a while, had been dismissed—as a gay problem. Conservatives can use fear to whip up homophobia, and liberals can use the conservatives' overreaction to expose what a threat conservatives are to minorities.

But the statistics may lie. The rate at which AIDS cases are doubling may be lower today than it was two-and-a-half years ago because fewer people are reporting the disease. Closet gays may not want the disease reported because they don't want their hidden life betrayed; doctors may not report the disease because they sympathize with the fears of closet-gay patients or because they simply don't have the time to do all the paperwork.

Everywhere I went, people said that the CDC's numbers were low for their city.

"Most of the cases I've seen," said a doctor at New York Hospital in Manhattan, "have not been reported."

In some small towns doctors might not even recognize AIDS.

As a social worker in Waco, Texas, said when confronted with a potential AIDS patient: "I can't believe this is AIDS. This is Waco. We have Baylor [University] here."

13.

Even if AIDS were spreading into the straight population at ten times the rate it does, fear and the resulting
panic would be a dangerous response. Fear feeds homophobia, encourages violence against gays, and promotes civil
liberties abuses. It creates pressure to quarantine those who
are sick or who are in risk groups and blows out of proportion issues like the question of where to house the sick and
whether or not kids with AIDS should be allowed to attend
public schools.

I'm not suggesting that we should not address serious
questions, like what to do with kids who have AIDS or how
to react to AIDS carriers who insist on being sexually active
and secretive about their condition. I'm suggesting that
these questions cannot be rationally addressed in a climate
of irrational fear.

Irrationality leads only to more irrationality. A hospital
in Virginia, had the affrontery to sue the mother of a baby
who died as a result of being given an AIDS-infected transfusion. Randy Lane, who had been arrested in Dade City,
Florida, for driving erratically, was released from jail when
the authorities found out he had AIDS. In fact the cops,
frantic to get rid of him, raised his bail and fine money and
put him on the road to Atlanta with a box lunch. And in a
hospital in Massachusetts, a desperate AIDS patient
stripped off his hospital gown and tried to commit suicide
by leaping from his window. His room was on a high floor;
he didn't know it was over a wing of the hospital that jutted
out only one story lower. He dropped a dozen feet and
landed, unhurt, on the roof of the annex, next to a coronary
ward. The heart attack patients who happened to be glanc-

ing out the window were confronted with a naked man pounding on the pane.

14.

In Denver, Carol Leese, the director of the Gay and Lesbian Community Center of Colorado, told me about a man who came home to die and who hadn't yet told his family he had AIDS, because he was afraid of being ostracized. And about a woman who bought an apartment from a gay man and decided to fumigate the place before she moved in.

In Boston, Larry Kessler of the AIDS project at the Fenway Community Health Center said they wanted a hot-line number that would spell out AIDS, "but New England Bell was not cooperative." Fear of AIDS is so high, the project even got a call from Cairo, Egypt, from a man who was worried that he might have picked up the disease from a Seattle, Washington, hooker.

In Chicago, AIDS patients were shunned in the hospitals. Nurses wouldn't enter the room; they'd leave food trays outside the door—something that also happened in other cities.

"We had some trouble with the staff," said a nurse in Hartford, Connecticut. "A lot of people don't want to work with anyone with AIDS. I will, but it can be a drag. The patient's friends sometimes cause trouble. I had to shave [the pubic hair of] one guy with AIDS. His friend got jealous. 'I can do that,' he said. I guess the one change in my habits is I won't eat finger food anymore."

In Jersey City, New Jersey, policemen refused to transport a prisoner whose brother was reported as having died of AIDS.

A major airline fired a gay flight attendant with swollen glands.

The United States Air Force wanted to deny medical benefits to a serviceman because it claimed catching AIDS was evidence of misconduct.

In San Antonio, policemen ordered anti-AIDS masks like the ones used for a short time in San Francisco.

In Houston, Texas, gay leaders "haven't had much contact with bath owners," said Michael Wilson of the KS/AIDS Foundation of Houston. "There's not much educational effort in the baths" going on.

In New York City, the state health department suggested that dentists wear special gowns, masks, gloves, and goggles when treating someone with AIDS—a precaution that some dentists don't find sufficient. In a poll of 350 Manhattan dentists, every one said he would not treat someone with AIDS and many said they wouldn't treat anyone who was gay. A gay doctor in his early thirties who developed Kaposi's in the early summer of 1982 lost his medical fellowship and was forced out of a job in a laboratory when his co-workers refused to work with him. In another poll last September in New York City, 42 percent wanted people with AIDS quarantined.

A new Colorado Board of Health decision demands a report of the name, address, age, and sex of anyone who has been exposed to AIDS.

Newark, New Jersey, and Dade County, Florida, are both considering laws requiring some sort of AIDS-free certification for food handlers. A candidate for mayor of New York said that under her administration the list of those who would need an AIDS-free guarantee would be expanded to include all doctors, nurses, teachers, and prostitutes.

The United States Navy refused a man treatment or an

honorable discharge unless he listed the people with whom he'd had sex.

West Germany has considered forced AIDS tests for people in risk groups and criminal sanctions against people with AIDS who have sex.

Outside the United States, researchers have so far identified about 3,000 AIDS cases in seventy-one countries. In one year, 1985, in Western Europe AIDS cases increased by 160 percent, doubling in the first eight months to 1,090. AIDS has begun appearing with greater frequency in France, Italy, Belgium, and Australia. Geneva and Paris now have about as many AIDS cases as Los Angeles. Hong Kong had its first case of AIDS in the summer of 1985. China has had one case—a visiting Argentinian. AIDS is flourishing in Cambodian refugee camps in Thailand. At least eight employees at the United Nations have AIDS; four have died, and the World Health Organization is now mobilizing against the disease.

In October 1985, Russia claimed to have no AIDS cases, but in the spring of 1985 there were reports of two cases, and in September UPI reported that Russian doctors admitted they had AIDS cases, caused by "mixed marriages," although no one explained what the term *mixed marriages* meant—men marrying men? marriages between different races? marriages between capitalists and communists?

Because of the increase of AIDS across the world, there is talk about restricting international travel of anyone not certifiably AIDS-free.

AIDS has become the monster in the closet, scaring us to sleep. It has justified a rising anxiety about sex among both heterosexuals and homosexuals, just as the fear of herpes did in the years before AIDS became a household word.

"America has used AIDS as an excuse to throw out the benefits of what we used to call the sexual revolution," said one gay man. "If AIDS never existed, we would have found something else to do the job."

At the birthday party of a friend's five-year-old, I talked to a doctor who has treated many people with AIDS.

"Our generation had the best of it," he said, "even if for only a short time. Drugs to cure syphilis and gonorrhea. The Pill—before we discovered the Pill could be fatal. We could run amok with sex, plunge into sex, explore it as if we were on some safe safari in a wildlife sanctuary. Get the thrill of seeing the prowling beasts but without the threat."

He gestured toward the boys and girls in the backyard who were doing the five-year-old's equivalent of flirting.

"What we've seen of AIDS is just the beginning," he said. "What do you think sex is going to be like for them when they grow up? God help them."

16.

"Early on," said Michael Callen, "a decision was made among the gay community to frighten the straight community"—presumably to galvanize the government into doing something about the epidemic. "I'm tremendously angry at how gays have marketed the disease."

By the time I'd made a circuit of AIDS centers around the country, I was discouraged by their apathy and frightened by the specter of an anti-AIDS backlash that could threaten the civil liberties of all gays—and, by extension, everyone in the country, gay or straight.

8 / A Quest for Salvation

Many centuries ago the Christians of Abyssinia saw in the plague a sure and God-sent means of winning eternal life. Those who were not yet stricken wrapped round them sheets in which men had died of plague, so as to make sure of their death. I grant you such a frenzied quest of salvation was not to be commended.

—Albert Camus,
The Plague

1.

JOEL Weisman, one of the first doctors in Los Angeles to treat AIDS patients, had talked about how much the gay community had denied AIDS, had refused to deal with it. When he talked publicly about it, "People told me, 'Cool it. You're creating homophobia.' "

But Weisman could not cool it.

"Having grown up in a Jewish background" with its history of oppression, Weisman said, "and having moved to California with its history of the Japanese internment," he doesn't believe one can stand silent when there is a danger that a minority might be persecuted by the majority.

Like Dr. Celso Bianco of the New York Blood Center and Larry Kramer, Weisman connects the reaction to AIDS to the extermination of Jews under Naziism.

"Concentration camps? I'd like to think that we, as Americans, are beyond that," he said, "but I don't think we are, as long as there are bigots and being gay is an issue. The potential is always there."

That's what worried him about the HTLV-3 test for AIDS promoted by Margaret Heckler and Robert Gallo and their colleagues.

"What does the test measure?" he asked. "Just exposure

is not good enough. What is the significance of the exposure?"

Does it mean you will get the disease? That you won't get the disease, but you're a carrier? Only that you had contact with someone who has the disease?

The CDC has refused to keep confidential the names of people reported to them as having AIDS.

"Homosexual sex is still a felony in twenty-three states," said Virginia Apuzzo, executive director of the National Gay Task Force. "How the hell do they expect us to answer questions like what drugs do we use and what do we do sexually? Where's this information going? Into whose computer bank? Do you want a list of ten million sick men who are also homosexual? I resisted the paranoia, but instinctive things go off in a crisis that make you remember you are not dealing with friendly institutions. It's a little like asking blacks in 1964 to trust labor unions that came to their assistance. *Thank you very much. Next!*"

2.

Every state has laws that can be used to isolate people with infectious diseases; and at least two states—California and Connecticut—have recently acted to change their laws to make the quarantining of people with AIDS easier.

In California Dr. James Chin, the chief of the state health department's Infectious Diseases Section, considered the possibility of enforced quarantine for anyone infected with AIDS who refused to "abstain from sexual activity that could transmit the AIDS agent" or who was "openly hostile" to recommendations of the health department. According to Robert Switzer, the president of Lawyers for Human Rights, quarantine in California had a precedent.

During the bubonic plague panic at the turn of the century, San Francisco created detention centers for the residents of Chinatown.

But Chin's suggestion was attacked and ridiculed—one commentator asked how the state would enforce the law: "Branding the sexual organs, 'Don't use me?' " And the state, at least for the time being, dropped the idea.

In Connecticut, a twenty-nine-year-old woman named Carlotta Locklear was arrested on charges of disorderly conduct when she tried to flag down a car near the corner of Chapel and Day streets, an area where hookers hang out. She'd been convicted fourteen times before on charges including prostitution and possession of heroin. Informers told authorities that people on the street thought she and her child, who was about one and a half years old, were AIDS carriers. In the Hospital of St. Raphael, where she was treated for pneumonia, she was kept in isolation. Anyone entering her room had to wear a special gown, surgical gloves, and a mask. She was taken to court by a guard wearing gloves, transported in a police van that was subsequently scrubbed out, and, to make sure she didn't walk out of the hospital as she had once before, strapped to her bed with rubber restraints.

"It boggles the mind that in 1984 a person would be treated that way," said her lawyer, John R. Williams.

The state wanted to make sure she was off the street and not infecting anyone.

Three other prostitutes suspected of having AIDS were also examined. And, although at the time the CDC claimed they didn't know of any cases in which a woman had infected a man with AIDS, three men who'd had sex with the hookers had symptoms of the disease.

"There's not a state facility besides an acute-care hospital willing to take an AIDS patient," said Dr. John Dwyer, former chief of immunology at Yale–New Haven Hospital, who examined some of the prostitutes. He felt the government had to set up special wards for people with AIDS.

"If the person [suspected of having AIDS] refuses to go," he said, "you need legislation to enforce it."

State Representative Richard Tulisano proposed an amendment to Connecticut's quarantine statute, which William Olds, the executive director of the Connecticut Civil Liberties Union, said could "sweep a person off the streets on mere suspicion."

In the spring of 1984 a revised version of the quarantine law passed both the state's House and Senate. It was signed by the governor on June 4 and became effective on October 1, 1984.

"I'm uncomfortable with it not so much for what it says as for what it doesn't say," said Dr. Alvin Novick, a professor of biology at Yale University and a co-chairman of the AIDS Project/New Haven. "Quarantine is such a devastating blow to someone's life. If it were invoked for someone with AIDS, it would forever after deprive them of job, social life, friends. It could be used as a statement of official oppression that is not unknown in our society, but that today is hardly tolerable. The people in public health are not precluded from being ignorant or evil. And there are people in public health who are evil and ignorant. There will be powerful spokespersons for such a move [to quarantine people with AIDS or suspected of having it]. Some of them will have the ear of the public."

3.

When the taxi driver saw that he was dropping me off at Denver's gay center, he said, "Shit. Faggots. Kikes. Niggers.

What's this country coming to. You offended? This ain't Jew York. Get out and walk."

In February 1984 *The Southern Medical Journal* published an editorial suggesting that AIDS was "a fulfillment of St. Paul's pronouncement: 'the due penalty' " for the error of men who " 'abandoned the natural function of the woman and burned in their desire toward one another. . . .' "

Last spring the right-wing American Life Lobby demanded the resignation of Assistant Secretary of Health Dr. Edward Brandt because he had announced he would present an award to a gay group for its extraordinary efforts "in the area of blood donations." The American Life Lobby called Brandt's participation in the ceremony an "outrageous legitimization of an unnatural life-style that is repugnant to the vast majority of Americans."

The *New Scientist* and *Nature,* both highly respected journals, ran articles on AIDS that conjured up Sodom and Gomorrah. And the piece in *Nature* went so far as to suggest that "male homosexuals should be persuaded to change their ways," a suggestion agreed to by an article in *The New England Journal of Medicine,* which advocated "taking appropriate measures to . . . 'rehabilitate' highly promiscuous homosexuals."

These recommendations may sound mild to the straight world—obviously in an epidemic people in a high-risk group should change their habits if it will prevent their infection. But the gay community remembers all too well theories about behavior modification that assumed homosexuality was a sickness; talk of *rehabilitation* is for gays what talk of *the final solution* is to survivors of Auchwitz.

In Dallas, Texas, Dallas Doctors Against AIDS have successfully fought to put sodomy laws back on the books and have tried to keep gay students from attending college, where they might somehow infect their classmates.

Homophobes view people with AIDS as aliens who, disguised as normal folk, are trying to take us over and are, like the invaders in H. G. Wells's *War of the Worlds,* dying because of an infection the "normal folk" are immune to.

Colorado is keeping a list of people exposed to AIDS. The San Antonio, Texas, City Health Department warned fourteen people with AIDS that if they had sex with anyone they could be charged with a felony.

The Moral Majority, Reverend Jerry Falwell's conservative organization, has asked for a national task force to draw up laws that would make it illegal for people with AIDS to have sex. And on May 20, 1985, Dr. James Mason, then director of the Centers for Disease Control, said that the Reagan Administration was considering quarantining people with AIDS.

In Seattle, Washington, teenage gangs armed with baseball bats and chains have terrorized the homosexual community in an anti-AIDS vigilante action that has been compared in ferocity to the Ku Klux Klan lynchings of blacks in the South.

In New York Hospital in March of 1984, a man with AIDS who was strapped to his bed for medical reasons was throttled by an intruder and set on fire.

"Usually the assailants want the victim to know the reason they're doing it is because he's queer," said Kevin Berrill, the coordinator of the National Gay Task Force Violence Project, which in an unprecedented study reported 1,682 incidents of "harassment, threats, and attacks" against homosexuals in the first eight months of 1984, the "same period," a National Gay Task Force statement said, "the gay community was hit by the first wave of violence attributed to 'AIDS backlash. . . .' AIDS was a motivating factor in nearly 20 percent of all incidents. . . ."

Between April and September of 1984 and the same pe-

riod in 1985, there was in San Francisco an 89 percent increase in violence against gays, much of it apparently due
to fear of AIDS. In the past year, the number of cases of
antigay violence reported to the New York City Human
Rights Commission has increased 100 percent.

The figure, Berrill said, may be only one-fifth of the actual number of cases.

"They want to kill us—all of us," said a gay man who
had just learned he had what may be a pre-AIDS condition.

4.

Every week I get letters from people with theories: *AIDS
has nothing to do with a virus or semen; it is caused by a parasite.
Or: AIDS affects only those who have been using antibiotics so frequently to fight off other sexually transmitted infections that their
systems no longer respond to medication. Or: Since, according to a
recent study reported in* Science, *sex hormones and the immune system are interrelated, perhaps gay men with atypical male sex hormone balances may be more prone to AIDS than others. Or: AIDS is
the result of being bombarded by strobe lights. Or: AIDS is an An-
dromeda strain brought down to earth by male aliens who on their
planet couple only with other males and who have infiltrated earth's
gay community.*

Conclusion: The Shadow of Death

A great scourge never appears unless there is a reason for it.

—Henry Miller,
The Air-Conditioned Nightmare

1.

AIDS is a paranoid's delight. So many theories. Such intricate possibilities. Almost from the start, nightmarish scenarios flourished.

Some believed the disease was a Frankenstein monster produced in some recombinant DNA lab and accidentally exposed to the world.

Others believed AIDS was part of a plot to kill off homosexuals. By the right wing. By the government. Gay men remind each other of instances of federal skullduggery like the experiments in the 1950s with LSD on unsuspecting subjects, and the Tuskegee Syphilis Experiment in which about four hundred poor black men suffering from syphilis were denied treatment so their progress could be studied by government-backed scientists. According to the *Washington Monthly* of July–August, 1985, for two decades—from the late 1940s to 1969—the United States Army, practicing for germ warfare, released what were assumed to be harmless microorganisms in various cities.

In 1969 a common bacterium, *Bacillus subtilis,* was released in the New York City subway system. The bacterium was also sprayed in the North Terminal of Washington, D.C.'s National Airport. Other secret experiments were carried out in California, Alaska, Florida, Panama City, and on the Pennsylvania Turnpike. Some of the biological warfare research was done at Ft. Detrick, near Frederick, Maryland.

There is a persistent rumor that AIDS was developed for biological warfare. One current version of this story claims that the virus was developed in the late 1970s at Ft. Detrick and was first tested in 1978, and that the project was named—appropriately, given the progress of AIDS—Operation Firm Hand.

The Russians, in the weekly magazine *Literaturnaya Gazeta,* claimed that the CIA developed AIDS and tested it on drunks and tramps in Haiti—a turnabout from their previous belief that AIDS was proof of the decadence of a capitalistic society.

"I think gay people have got to see themselves as being murdered," said Chuck Ortleb, publisher of *New York Native,* who believes AIDS is a human version of an animal disease: African swine fever, which suppresses the immune system of pigs and causes pneumonia, various other opportunistic infections, and a disease similar to Kaposi's sarcoma. (It is especially prevalent, according to Dr. C. Prakash of Ohio State University Agricultural Research and Development Center, among male pigs that exhibit homosexual activity.) The African swine fever virus is present in blood, semen, urine—as the AIDS virus (if it is a virus) seems to be. And outbreaks of African swine fever have occurred simultaneously with outbreaks of AIDS in Haiti and Zaire (which has a special trade relationship with Haiti).

"The parallels [between the two diseases] are overwhelming," Ortleb said.

Although Dr. Don Francis, the assistant director of the CDC's Division of Viral Diseases, has said, "You won't find more than four scientists in the whole world who adhere to that [the African swine fever] theory," Dr. Jane Teas, a scientist who once worked at the Harvard School of Public Health, noted the coincidence between the two diseases. The Commonwealth of Pennsylvania House of Representatives cited her "pioneering efforts . . . in linking the cause of AIDS possibly to the . . . African swine fever virus."

In the March 8th, 1986, issue of *The Lancet*, Jane Teas, John Beldekas of Boston University, and James Herbert of the American Health Foundation published the results of research that found evidence of African Swine Fever Virus in the blood of nearly 50 percent of the people with AIDS who were tested.

In January of 1977 the *Boston Globe* reported: "With at least the tacit backing of U.S. Central Intelligence Agency officials, operatives linked to anti-Castro terrorists introduced African swine fever virus into Cuba in 1971. . . ."

A U.S. intelligence source leaked to *Newsday* that "he was given the virus in a sealed, unmarked container at a U.S. Army base and CIA training ground in the Panama Canal Zone [Ft. Gutlick], with instructions to turn it over to the anti-Castro group."

The outbreak of African swine fever in 1971 marked the disease's introduction to the Western hemisphere. The virus spread to Haiti, the Dominican Republic, and Brazil.

If AIDS is African swine fever, and if African swine fever was imported to our part of the world by the CIA, what possibilities for a grand conspiracy theory! *Gays begin to come out of the closet and seize their rights in society; reactionaries in power panic and think of a plot to prevent what they see is the feminization—or effeminization—of American culture!*

But the explanation for AIDS probably doesn't involve any conspiracy more sinister than the one played on us by nature. AIDS is most likely caused by HTLV-3/LAV, a virus from Africa, acting with particular host factors, like semen or drugs, which impair the immune system. The test for exposure to AIDS will not be misused by the government, and there will soon be a vaccine to protect us against the disease. There may even be cures—like Dapsone or Interferon, HPA-23, or a glandular extract (like the one used in Israel to treat AIDS), Azidothymidine, Ribavirin, Suramin, or some other scientific wonder—for the opportunistic infections and Kaposi's sarcoma and the primary disease itself. It will all turn out to be very innocent. Very simple.

The great London plague was caused by the city's communal pump. They stopped using the pump, and the plague went away.

2.

I'll end with a cautionary tale.

The bubonic plague began in the foothills of the Himalayas in a region known as Garwhal and Kumaon. The Saracen empire acted as a buffer to protect Europe from the disease. So when the Europeans fought the Saracens during the Crusades, the more successful they were on the battlefield, the more vulnerable they were making themselves to the disease at home.

The moral? Be careful what battles you win.